ILLNESS IS A WEAPON

ILLNESS IS A WEAPON

Indigenous Identity and Enduring Afflictions

Eirik Saethre

Vanderbilt University Press

Nashville

This book is printed on acid-free paper.
Manufactured in the United States of America

Library of Congress Cataloging-in-Publication Data on file

LC control number 2012033912
LC classification number RA553.S236 2012
Dewey class number 362.1089'99—dc23

ISBN 978-0-8265-1920-7 (cloth)
ISBN 978-0-8265-1922-1 (e-book)

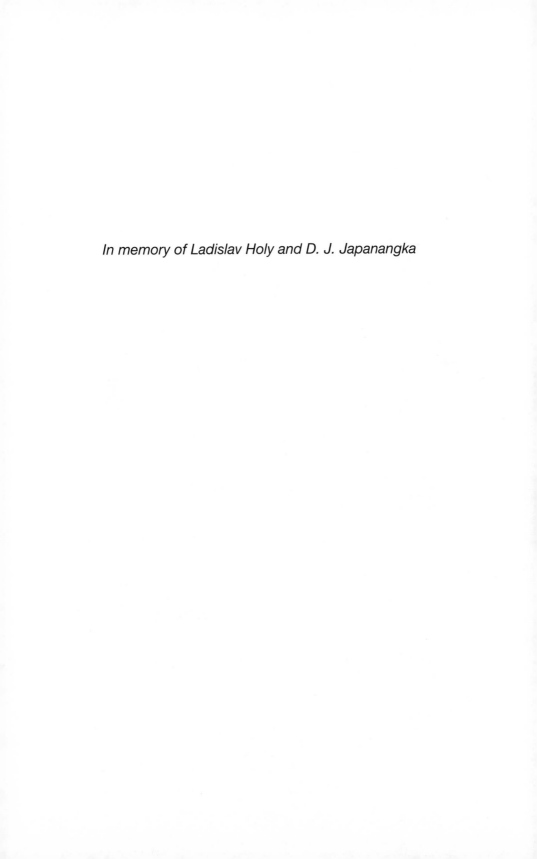

In memory of Ladislav Holy and D. J. Japanangka

Contents

Acknowledgments

This book would not have been possible without the support and guidance of a number of individuals. Foremost, I would like to thank the Warlpiri people of Lajamanu who brought me into their families, taught me how to hunt, took me to ceremony, and always looked after me. I must also recognize the invaluable assistance of the medical staff of the Lajamanu Community Health Centre. While there are many names I could list, I will refrain from doing so to protect the privacy of individuals who appear in this book.

For assisting with the creation and completion of this project as a PhD thesis at the Australian National University, I would like to thank Nicolas Peterson, Margot Lyon, Francesca Merlan, Yasmine Musharbash, Katie Glaskin, Derek Elias, Goran Sevo, and Roberta James. I must also acknowledge the financial support of the Australian National University and the Australian Institute of Aboriginal and Torres Strait Islander Studies.

For providing unerring guidance as I transformed the thesis into a book, I must thank Isak Niehaus, John Sharp, Geoffrey White, Christine Yano, and Christine Beaule.

CHAPTER 1
Everyday Illness

In Australia's outback, disease and suffering have become a part of the everyday lives of Aboriginal people. On a recent visit to Lajamanu, a Warlpiri community in the Northern Territory, I was reminded that illness is ubiquitous and often taken for granted. For residents such as Martin, sicknesses, fevers, aches, and pains are now an accepted feature of their existence.[1] When we first met in 1997, Martin was working regularly, but after several years of ill health, he became unemployed and reliant on government assistance payments. During a recent conversation with Martin, I noticed several large scars covering his abdomen, the result of repeated surgeries. Looking gaunt and with his bones clearly visible, I asked how long he had been this thin. Pleased, Martin replied that he had gotten "up to" his normal weight. I was surprised that Martin considered his current appearance to be unremarkable. When we first met, he looked very different. While not a large man, photos of Martin from my early days in Lajamanu show him with a round face and a slightly protruding stomach. Given the dramatic change in his appearance, I asked how he was feeling. Martin told me he had been experiencing almost constant pain for several years. I expressed concern over his chronic poor health and asked what treatments had been prescribed. Annoyed that I could not see the obvious, Martin replied that his health was not poor. Although he had been ill a few years ago, Martin assured me that he was now in "excellent health." He added, "I don't have anything anymore. I'm right [healthy]." After a moment, almost as an afterthought, he added, "I have that sugar one [diabetes] but everyone has that. So that really doesn't matter."

Martin was not exceptional. Despite living in a wealthy nation with a comprehensive health infrastructure, Indigenous Australians—Aboriginal people and Torres Strait Islanders—endure a high burden of disease.[2] Epidemiological data clearly reveals the magnitude of ill health. The average national life expectancy is 59 years for Indigenous males and 65 years for Indigenous females (Pink and Allbon 2008, 5). This is

1

five years below the global average and comparable to life expectancy in Bangladesh, Mauritania, and Turkmenistan (United Nations 2007, 79, 80). Furthermore, these statistics are not improving. Over the past thirty years, Indigenous groups across the country have yet to see a noticeable reduction in rates of ill health (Public Accounts Committee 1996, 63; Ring and Brown 2002, 630). In some areas, Indigenous health is worsening. Between 2001 and 2005, rates of heart disease, circulatory problems, diabetes, and kidney diseases all increased (Pink and Allbon 2008, 104). As the years progress, the disparity between Indigenous and non-Indigenous health in Australia is widening.

The Northern Territory is the epicenter of this epidemic. Speaking with Aboriginal people, one is struck by the numerous tales of scabies, boils, diarrhea, trachoma, diabetes, rheumatic heart disease, hypertension, heart attacks, amputations, and strokes. Martin's comment that "everyone" has diabetes reflects the seeming ubiquity of ill health. Statistics indicate that Aboriginal Territorians have the dubious distinction of possessing the lowest life expectancy in the country (Australian Bureau of Statistics 2009). On average, they will live approximately twenty years less and have a burden of disease 2.5 times higher than that of a non-Aboriginal Territorian (Northern Territory Department of Health 2004, 24; Zhao et al. 2004). Although Indigenous mortality and morbidity rates increase appreciably in the remote regions of the continent, this cannot be attributed solely to a lack of medical facilities.[3] In Lajamanu, the clinic provides medical care and distributes prescription pharmaceuticals free of charge. Patients requiring more comprehensive treatments are flown to the hospital in Katherine, also at no cost. Not only are medical services supplied, they are utilized. On an average day, staff of the Lajamanu Community Health Centre treat a significant proportion of the population—around 7 percent—much higher than in the urban areas of the country. While some individuals utilize the clinic more regularly than others, many residents consult medical staff several times over the course of a year. Despite receiving care, health remains poor.

Indigenous health disparities are not unique to Australia. Around the world, Indigenous populations consistently suffer from higher rates of illness (Ferreira and Lang 2006). Even though countries such as Australia, Canada, New Zealand, and the United States have funded health interventions and introduced dedicated treatment facilities, the health of their Indigenous peoples continues to lag behind national averages. These trends are rooted in longstanding relationships between Indigenous people, non-Indigenous settlers, and illness. The European conquest of the Americas and Oceania is thought to have been greatly assisted by the introduction of previously unknown infectious diseases including influenza, chicken pox, and measles. In some instances—such as stories of blankets infested with smallpox—it seems as if purposeful infection occurred as an early form of germ warfare. While pathogens were taking their toll on Indigenous people, concerns that the white population was vulnerable to contagion were invoked as justification to quarantine and segregate Indigenous people on reservations.

Although Indigenous people have subsequently achieved greater rights and access to improved medical care, earlier trends have not been completely reversed. Many Indigenous people continue to live on remote or undesirable land and have lower levels of income and education than do non-Indigenous people. Furthermore, diseases considered to have been introduced by white colonizers still afflict Indigenous populations. As influenza disparately affected Indigenous communities in the past, diabetes and other chronic diseases—often considered to be the result of consuming "white" or introduced commercial foods—are taking a heavy toll on contemporary generations. Consequently, illness and the marginalization of Indigenous people have become inexorably linked. Transcending epidemiological data regarding morbidity and mortality, understandings about, and responses to, Indigenous ill health are embedded within current debates about European settlement, race relations, and Indigeneity.

Through medical dialogues, the "long conversation" between colonizers and colonized is continued (Comaroff and Comaroff 1991). Disease and medicine have been, and continue to be, powerful ways of explaining the world. Medical narratives often reflect social ones, particularly in colonial and post-colonial environments (Bibeau and Pedersen 2002; Crandon-Malamud 1993; Langford 2002; Marshall 2005; Roy 2006; Treichler 1999). These social meanings become particularly evident in epidemics, which Fassin (2007, 32) characterizes as "moments of truth when both knowledge and power are put to the test." Uncovering rather than inventing, epidemics create a space through which social beliefs and attitudes are laid bare. Furthermore, medical narratives and interventions aimed at eradicating health inequalities can play a pivotal role in articulating an identity for Indigenous citizens, while actually creating the conditions that they sought to improve (Briggs and Mantini-Briggs 2003). It is not a coincidence that the history of epidemics and the history of racism often coincide.

In Australia—where Aboriginal ill health has also been dubbed an epidemic—Indigenous identity has become inextricably tied to disease (Kowal and Paradies 2010, 599). On one hand, health statistics and campaigns reinforce the link between disease and Indigeneity. On the other, Aboriginal responses that dismiss the exceptionality of illness—such as Martin's statement that diabetes "doesn't matter"—have led some medical staff to refer to Aboriginal people as "irresponsible," "uncaring," and "noncompliant," further entrenching existing notions of Indigenous Otherness. Remarking on the "aetiological opacity of chronic disease," Lea (2008, 135-136) notes, "As the visual image may lack the look of disease, and fail to enact the performative dimension of unwellness, the asymptomatically diseased Indigenous body cannot be trusted to tell an immediately ascertainable story." Instead, a story is created that draws from pervasive and persistent notions of culture, race, personhood, and citizenship. Through an exploration of narratives, beliefs, and practices surrounding ill health, the construction and maintenance of Indigenous identities—as well as the conditions that make these identities possible—are made manifest.

Responding to governmental and medical explanations, Indigenous people fashion their own narratives. Warlpiri tales of illness and treatment continually portray Aboriginal people as suffering physically and socially as a result of inadequate care, racist medical staff, and oppressive government control. Although Martin spoke of diabetes as unexceptional, he commented, "If we were *kardiya* [white people] living in a *kardiya* [white] community we would be treated right. We would be healthy." Complaints of chronic illness and mistreatment during care are marshalled as evidence to motivate "talking back." Over a decade ago, I spoke to Catherine after she had returned from taking her two-year-old daughter, Joyce, for medical tests at the hospital in town. At the time, Catherine told me the hospital visit was an unwarranted imposition, complaining that non-Aboriginal nurses believed that Aboriginal people are unable to care for their children properly and so order unnecessary tests. Catherine said, "[The nurses] are racist. That is why they make [Aboriginal people] get checked so much when nothing is wrong." Unhappy at the treatment that she and her daughter had received, Catherine recounted her response during Joyce's exam. When medical staff speculated that Joyce's silence could indicate a learning disability, Catherine replied, "She can talk. She can say 'fuck you.'"

Recently, I asked Catherine how her daughter was doing. Catherine answered nonchalantly, "She is fine. Those nurses were wrong. She only has kidney failure." Although Catherine was told that Joyce might soon need dialysis, she remained skeptical. Catherine said, "They don't know really." As proof, she commented that her son had suffered from "lung problems" as a child and an inability to breathe properly, but "grew out of them" during puberty. As had others, Catherine expressed dissatisfaction with the medical treatment she received from non-Aboriginal people. Describing how she was "forced" to have a portion of her thyroid removed, Catherine commented, "They treat us like we are animals." After a moment, Catherine added that, like her children, she also had also suffered repeated health crises throughout her life. Being Warlpiri, according to Catherine, meant being sick.

Although often synonymous with subjugation, I believe that sickness can also be a tool of confrontation. In an environment of pervasive racial disparity, disease is an idiom and an identity through which Indigenous people are able to actively argue for recognition and rights. As Indigeneity becomes associated with illness, being sick is an embodied tool of contestation as well as an effective strategy of resistance. Cursing at nurses, refusing to take medication, and accepting acute illness as unremarkable are simultaneously acts of defiance and rejections of vulnerability. Through a reexamination of the relationship among illness, identity, and race relations, this book asserts that disease and suffering are vigorous expressions of Indigeneity and, as a result, powerful methods of protest. Experiences of, and responses to, illness reflect not only the tactics individuals use to negotiate everyday realities but also a dialogue that constructs, manages, and challenges social relations.

Race, Culture, and Medicine

Medicine has been, and continues to be, a vehicle through which social identities are generated and managed. In his investigation of the creation of teaching hospitals in late eighteenth century Europe, Foucault (1973) charts the rise of the medical gaze in dominating a range of social institutions, ultimately acting as a tool for governing bodies. In part, the creation of medical and scientific epistemologies regarding the human condition grew out of encounters with the non-European world (Comaroff 1993, 308). Colonial ideas depicting the savagery and pathology of local populations became medical ones as popular notions of nature and difference were translated into scientific discourse. In the early nineteenth century, Georges Cuvier argued that physiological differences in cranial shape placed the "negro" between Europeans and the "most ferocious apes" (Figlio 1976, 28). Prior to the advent of bacteriology, colonial missionaries described African bodies as radiating contagion and noxious organisms—an "infested 'greasy' native—indistinguishable from the pestilential surroundings" (Comaroff 1993, 316).

Medicine reinforced conceptual boundaries between Europeans and non-Europeans while also serving as a tool that encouraged and extended colonization. A permanent and long-term European presence was required in the tropics to effectively sustain trade and establish colonial governments. Driven by a need to decrease the high rates of European mortality in the equatorial regions, tropical medicine was developed as a "fundamentally imperialistic" discipline (Farley 1991, 3). Throughout the British-dominated world, the expansion of medicine was linked to the expansion of colonial interests. The London School of Tropical Medicine was effectively a medical department of the colonial office in its early years (Worboys 1990, 25). Ostensibly justified as a concern for public health, medicine was invoked by colonial officials and settlers to control local populations. For instance, the British only began addressing illness affecting Indians as a result of the need to systematically rule the subcontinent politically and militarily (Arnold 1993, 24). South Africa's first national health measure and one that would remain in place until 1977, the Public Health Act (1919), advocated racial segregation as a means of arresting the spread of disease (Phillips 1990). Throughout the interwar years, as black migration to white urban centers increased, health officials argued that a large metropolitan black population would lead to poor sanitation and increased illness rates, thus justifying stricter influx controls (Comaroff and Comaroff 1992, 229; Jochelson 2001).

In Australia, researchers have similarly stressed the links among tropical medicine, public health, and race within the colonial context (Anderson 2006; Gillespie 1991; Harloe 1991; Walker 1997/98; Yarwood 1991). The susceptibility of Aboriginal people to introduced diseases was often invoked as a metaphor for understanding racial relations. A lack of resistance to illnesses was equated to a lack of resistance to colonization (Bashford 2000, 258). Due in part to a high mortality rate, from the 1850s to the 1930s, Aboriginal people were viewed as a "doomed race" destined to become extinct. Casting Aboriginal people as primitive hunters and gatherers, these views invoked the "science" of evolution to argue that Aboriginal people were unable to adapt to the modern world, while ignoring the devastating impact of colonialism and settlement (McGregor 1997).

Non-Aboriginal people used Aboriginal responses to medicine and disease to create notions of Aboriginal agency and morality. In an effort to understand Aboriginal physiology, a number of medical expeditions were made during the first half of the twentieth century by men like John Burton Cleland. While Aboriginal people were repeatedly subjected to medical tests, researchers often remarked on Aboriginal passivity to white intrusion (Thomas 2004, 78). Aboriginal subjects were cast as good-natured but inert. In addition, disparate rates of disease, particularly introduced sexually transmitted diseases, created and reinforced ideas of Aboriginality. Their prevalence led these diseases to be labeled the "black pox" or "Native pox" (O'Brien 1998). Because of their association with sexually transmitted diseases, Aboriginal people were considered to lack morality, restraint, and other important and "civilizing" social skills.

As in South Africa and elsewhere, public health initiatives were employed to monitor and control Indigenous bodies. Bashford (2000, 258) notes, "Aboriginal people were often managed *through* health measures; that is, the 'race problem' was not infrequently thinly veiled as the 'health problem.'" In an effort to arrest the spread of leprosy, a number of health policies were enacted that severely restricted the movement of Aboriginal people. Prior to 1949 in the Kimberly region, leprosy "hunts" would often forcefully remove "troublemakers" from settlements under the guise of public health (Jebb 2002). In the Northern Territory, Aboriginal people who had contracted leprosy were taken to Darwin in neck chains (Rose 1991). From 1941 until 1963 a "leper line" was established along the twentieth parallel and Aboriginal residents were barred from travelling south of this boundary (Hunter 1993). Although justified using the language of health, relocations were designed to remove opposition to settlement and to exploit Aboriginal labor.

On the eve of World War II the Australian government began adopting a policy of assimilation whereby Aboriginal people were to be taught—and eventually adopt—the practices and values of white settler society (Beckett 2010). Government officials viewed hygiene and medical compliance as tools to accomplish this goal. The hope was that Aboriginal people would learn to become model citizens through the discipline of health behavior. In many instances Aboriginal people were coerced into following medical protocols established by the government. Nursing staff in the Northern Territory instructed police to collect "unreliable" patients and bring them to the clinic (Taylor 1978, 41). Upon presentation, a nurse ensured that the appropriate medication was ingested before allowing the individual to return home. Adherence to medical protocols quickly became a measure to gauge the level of Aboriginal assimilation into mainstream society. Consequently, health status and citizenship became linked. The Native Act of 1944 granted Australian citizenship to some Aboriginal people, but excluded those that were "full-bloods" and those with leprosy, syphilis, granuloma, and yaws—diseases which were considered a sign of poor morality and closely associated with Aboriginal communities (Mitchell 2007, 51). The certificate of citizenship could be revoked if these illnesses were later contracted by successful applicants.

By the end of the 1960s, the policy of assimilation was being abandoned. The legal status of Aboriginal people changed from wards of the Australian state to full citizens. Aboriginal practices that were once viewed as primitive and systematically discouraged under a policy of assimilation were being reevaluated in parallel with the shift in social status. Rather than dismissed as mere superstition, the health beliefs of Indigenous Australians were now conceptualized in terms of a medical system: an integrated structure of notions and practices that assisted in maintaining stable social relations. Anthropologists and researchers such as Berndt (1964), Cawte (1965; 1974), Eastwell (1973), Gray (1979), and Taylor (1977) all embrace this approach. For the first time, Aboriginal health beliefs were considered in their own right, although these authors often assumed, as did many others, that biomedical practitioners would eventually replace local Aboriginal healers. Similar to earlier views, Indigenous beliefs and practices were portrayed as largely distinct from, and unrelated to, those of non-Aboriginal Australians. This approach relied on the assumption that Aboriginal people—particularly those living in the remote regions of the continent, such as the Northern Territory—possessed a unique cultural heritage that was derived from their collective existence as hunters and gatherers prior to the colonization of Australia. Contemporary contexts such as segregation, poverty, and racial conflict were largely ignored in favor of the traditional.

By the 1980s and 1990s, authors such as Devanesen (1985), Mobbs (1991), Nathan and Leichleitner (1983), and Reid (1983), continued to highlight the importance and uniqueness of Aboriginal beliefs and practices. The Indigenous health system was characterized as holistic and social, while biomedicine was cast as mechanical and alienating. This led some researchers and medical professionals to assert that Aboriginal health was not improving because biomedical care was culturally unsuited to Aboriginal populations. Continued instances of chronic illness, for example, were attributed partly to the "deep cultural gap" that was thought to exist between Aboriginal people and medical professionals (Devitt and McMasters 1998, 164). Failures to improve Aboriginal health were cast as failures to understand or respect Aboriginal worldviews, leading to calls for culturally appropriate care. Government initiatives in the Northern Territory such as "two way" medicine, the Aboriginal Health Worker Program, and community controlled health centers were designed to acknowledge Aboriginal beliefs and ways of life. These programs reflected the persistent belief that biomedical and Aboriginal systems of health were divergent, incommensurable, and conflicting.

More recently, anthropologists have paid greater attention to situating health beliefs within everyday social worlds. In examining Aboriginal health in rural New South Wales, Heil (2009) argues that we must shift from Western ideas of "embodied selves" to Aboriginal ideas of "social selves" to understand the way in which Aboriginal people conceive of well-being. These social selves are created and maintained through interpersonal exchanges and acts of sharing. Heil and Macdonald (2008, 301) contend that Aboriginal people differ in outlook from Westerners for whom the individual, not the collective, holds pride of place. Heil (2006, 107) writes, "In regard to clinical encounters between health staff and Aboriginal patients, the issue is *not* that these parties have different understandings and expectations of 'health' in conventional biomedical terms. They have different understandings and expectations of life as they experience it—and these often seem to be so much a world apart that the conjunctures in understandings of health cannot be bridged in the arena of treatment."

Widespread assertions that Australia's Indigenous people are culturally exceptional have led to calls for self-determination. The foundations of self-determination rest on what Kowal (2010, 189) terms a "post-colonial logic" that

> includes the belief that Indigenous culture is spiritually, socially, and ecologically superior to western culture in many ways; that the dispossession of Indigenous people and the destruction of much Indigenous culture is the cause of social and health problems in Indigenous

communities, and that the Australian people and their governments must accept responsibility for the injuries inflected on Indigenous people and cultures and invest more resources in Indigenous programs that are controlled by Indigenous people themselves.

As a result, Indigenous health has become one of the most politicized issues in the nation. Rather than simply a physical condition brought about by poor nutrition or hygiene, illness is linked to colonialism, dispossession, poverty, social exclusion, racism, assimilation, and paternalism (Flick and Nelson 1994; Tatz 1972; Tyler 1993). For some, the solution to the epidemic was not improved medical services, but land rights and Aboriginal control of resources. Flick and Nelson (1994, 5) write that Aboriginal health will not be resolved by improving the clinical issues, but by addressing the feelings of powerlessness and psycho-social or spiritual disease which currently afflict Aboriginal people. Government goals of achieving statistical parity between Aboriginal and non-Aboriginal rates of disease have been cast as a moral project intended to homogenize and assimilate the Aboriginal population (Tyler 1992, 17). Building upon the assumption that Western and Aboriginal traditions were incommensurable, biomedicine was seen as the problem, not the solution.

At the beginning of the twenty-first century the policy of self-determination began to be challenged. A neoliberal agenda emerged that sought to encourage social equality by discouraging cultural difference (Lattas and Morris 2010; Povenelli 2010). Culture was not the solution; it was part of the problem. Poor health is no longer portrayed as resulting exclusively from white intervention, Aboriginal exclusion, and cultural loss. Instead, the continued existence of beliefs and practices considered to be uniquely Aboriginal are also implicated. Neoliberal perspectives are perhaps best encapsulated in Sutton's (2009) *The Politics of Suffering*, a controversial book that has been both praised and vilified. Sutton argues that years of self-determination have not led to significant improvements in Aboriginal health, education, income, or other important indicators. Sutton (2009, 84) writes, "What is repeatedly missing in officialese accounts of what lies behind 'disadvantage' is the very thing that everyone in such circles is usually quick to say needs proper recognition—Indigenous tradition, social values and culture." To illustrate his point, Sutton blames poor health and hygiene on habits learned from hunting and gathering as well as the demand sharing of food, belief in sorcery, and a propensity for personal autonomy. He believes that improved health entails adopting new ways of life, not valorizing traditional ones. Reflecting on the activities of missionaries who coercively trained Aboriginal people to boil their sheets, Sutton (2009, 132) opines, "On health grounds one would have to say that whether imposed from outside, or adopted as people's own practice, this kind of assimilation, given the biological facts of the settled life, was not a calamity; it was a necessity." Seeking to resist the overt politicization of health in Australia—where high rates of morbidity and mortality are blamed almost solely on colonization and social inequality—Sutton draws attention to the agency and actions of Indigenous people. Although ostensibly opposed to the assumptions of self-determination, Sutton nevertheless shares one of its beliefs: Ill health is the result of the clash between old and new "health cultures."

Over the past several years, neoliberal policies have garnered increasing support in the Australian government. The most dramatic example occurred in 2007 when the Commonwealth government suspended the Racial Discrimination Act (1975) and enacted the Northern Territory Emergency Response. The Intervention, as it is popularly called, was motivated by a government report, *Ampe Akelyernemane Meke Mekarle "Little Children Are Sacred"* (Board of Inquiry into the Protection of Aboriginal Children from Sexual Abuse 2007). This report documented widespread child sexual abuse in Aboriginal communities. The Intervention significantly restructured life for many Aboriginal Territorians. The number of police officers stationed in remote communities increased. The permit system, which required non-Aboriginal people to obtain permission before entering Aboriginal land, was suspended. Aboriginal local government was reorganized. The bulk of welfare payments to Aboriginal people were placed into managed accounts, where they could only be withdrawn to purchase approved items at specified shops. Defending its decision to enact racially discriminatory legislation, the government argued that the Intervention was needed to end child sexual abuse, improve overall child health, and close the health gap between Aboriginal and non-Aboriginal Territorians. In their critical examination of these claims, Lattas and Morris (2010, 62) write, "Today, in the Northern Territory, what seems like a return to old disciplinary and paternalistic racial regimes can be understood as experiments in neoliberal forms of governmentality, which deny their racist character by formulating themselves as economical, necessary forms of practical care in exceptional circumstances." As the Intervention progressed, community clinics were tapped to play a greater role in monitoring the behavior of Aboriginal residents (Board of Inquiry into the Protection of Aboriginal Children from Sexual Abuse 2007, 136). Intimately tied to health status and medical service provision, the Intervention reinforced the relationships among government control, medicine, and race.

From the introduction of colonial medicine and through assimilation, self-determination and neoliberalism, notions of difference have been repeatedly marshaled to define, understand, and manage Aboriginal people. Although the explicitly racial theories of the nineteenth century are often dismissed as an unfortunate consequence of a remote past, their specter continues to linger in the concept of culture. Culture is often employed as an acceptable homologue for race in explaining human variation (Kuper 1999; Malik 1996; Stocking 1982). Beginning in the 1960s earlier Australian notions of race were transformed into beliefs regarding culture as "full-blooded." Aboriginal people began to be described as "traditional," whereas "half-castes" or "mixed-bloods" were "non-traditional" (Cowlishaw 1986, 3). Culture became a worldwide medium through which differences could be justified, despite its early use as a method to challenge racial theories in the United States. Macleod and Durrheim (2002, 788) comment, "In the place of biological 'scientific' racism, we have a 'new racism' in which 'culture,' 'tradition' and 'ethnicity' perform the work previously achieved by the category of 'race.'" By stressing the differences rather than the similarities between people, culture provided an explanation for the variation among peoples by supplying a mechanism through which beliefs and habits could be transferred relatively unchanged from one generation to the next.

For the past several decades in Australia a popular culture narrative has drawn from assumptions of difference and permeated the national consciousness. As in many of the instances in which the culture concept is invoked, it is used ideologically rather than anthropologically (Peterson 2010, 253). The culture narrative includes four assumptions:

1. The actions and beliefs of Aboriginal people are primarily and fundamentally based in, and driven by, culture.
2. Culture is the result of a continuation of beliefs and practices that existed prior to contact with the West.
3. Aboriginal people living in remote regions have stronger links to this past than do those living in urban areas.
4. Aboriginal culture is fundamentally different from non-Aboriginal culture.

The culture narrative, like the race narrative before it, is a product of a history of interactions that has resulted in the creation and maintenance of divergent identities. It also provides a convenient justification for Aboriginal disadvantage. But as Farmer (2003, 48) observes, culture does not explain suffering; "it may at worst furnish an alibi."

The culture concept is often invoked in discussions of Indigenous health. When examining the role of culture in health behavior, researchers tend to assume that black and Indigenous individuals are motivated by culture in a way that white people are not (Briggs and Mantini-Briggs 2003; Macleod and Durrheim 2002). Culture is often essentialized, cast as static, conflated with racial or ethnic categories, and then blamed for health disparities (Carpenter-Song, Schwallie, and Longhofer 2007; Kleinman and Benson 2006a; Santiago-Irizarry 2001; Taylor 2003). In sub-Saharan Africa, the HIV pandemic was thought to be the result of African cultural practices, such as promiscuity and dry sex (Caldwell, Caldwell, and Quiggin 1989; Stillwaggon 2003; Saethre and Stadler 2009). In Venezuela, Indigenous food and hygiene practices were condemned when a cholera epidemic struck the nation (Briggs and Mantini-Briggs 2003). While routinely portrayed as culture-free, biomedicine is thought to provide efficacious solutions—pharmaceuticals, medical technology, and best practice protocols—to combat the health threats posed by local beliefs. Consequently, biomedicine has been characterized as a "culture of no culture" (Taylor 2003).

While the solution to Aboriginal ill health is hotly debated between those supporting self-determination and those advocating intervention, all sides seem to agree that a fundamental difference exists between Aboriginal and non-Aboriginal people. Furthermore, it is this difference that is responsible for continued ill health. Culture is transformed into an agent that prevents *us* from helping *them*, whether it is because *we* do not understand *their* culture or because *their* culture is not adaptable to *our* technologies. Invoking culture in this manner can significantly constrain understandings of, and responses to, Aboriginal ill health. Humphery (2006) warns that reifying and exaggerating the role of culture can lead to "culture blindness," where other important factors that have an impact on the lives of Aboriginal people are ignored. This book will explore those factors in an attempt to move away from perspectives that exclusively employ culture as an explanatory device.

In posing a critical response to the popular culture narrative, I do not intend to question the fact that difference does exist. Aboriginal people do possess a unique history, worldview, cosmology, and identity. Invoking the culture narrative as the *primary* or *only* explanation for Aboriginal beliefs and actions, however, ignores the jumble of everyday life. Researchers have tended to focus on Aboriginal people as isolated, rather than acknowledging that they live side-by-side with non-Aboriginal people, with whom they interact on a daily basis (Cowlishaw 2010, 52). Although these engagements have at times been examined, in many instances the continuity and distinctiveness of Aboriginal traditions are emphasized. Collmann (1988, 227) notes, "The wider historical processes that have totally reorganized Aboriginal residence and work patterns in the twentieth century are used only as analytic screen through which to filter the modern data in order to sift their impact and leave an authentic customary residue." Rather than reifying culture, custom, or tradition and using these concepts as a tool to provide a blanket explanation for Aboriginal exceptionalism, I intend to shift the focus to contemporary sociality and experience.

In contrast to anthropological approaches that stress the continuation and uniqueness of Aboriginal customs, labeled "tradition" or "classism," other perspectives that are dubbed "modern blackness" or "interculturalism" focus on the ways in which ongoing racial relationships shape the lives and identities of Aboriginal people (Austin-Broos 2009, 12; Hinkson 2010, 5). For Merlan (2005, 167), interculturalism constitutes an examination of "the forms of engagement and influence between Aboriginal and non-Aboriginal people and institutions, and the implications of this for change." Rather than being seen as simply culturally different, Cowlishaw (2010, 57) believes that Aboriginal people should be viewed as "part of the Australian nation in particular circumstances." The intercultural perspective does not contest the notion of boundaries; instead, it seeks to explain how difference is contextualized and tactically negotiated in everyday life (Sullivan 2005, 2006). In so doing, it illuminates the ways in which present political circumstances have shaped understandings of the past, culture, and tradition. I wish to draw from this perspective and investigate Aboriginal health beliefs and practices as a product of ongoing social relationships within the contemporary Australian nation state.

Examining land rights legislation, Correy (2006) argues that that the claim process itself has helped to create the category of "traditional owner." The legal criteria for traditional ownership have shaped attitudes and beliefs regarding Aboriginality. Correy (2006, 337) writes, "This establishes traditional ownership as a sort of social category that then concretises the social groups it constructs. These groups have a social and political reality that is largely determined by the style and imagination of the discourse itself." Much like land rights legislation, medical policies and interventions also create an Aboriginal identity. From the earliest encounters between Aboriginal people and the white government, notions of Aboriginality were generated and entrenched through narratives of the "black pox," medical systems, and the pathology of Aboriginal ways of life. Rather than simply describing and treating disease, medicine has fashioned Aboriginality and continues to do so. Medical concerns regarding the health "gap" or Indigenous "noncompliance" powerfully and persuasively shape conceptions of Aboriginal identity. As medical topics are featured ever more frequently in the media and popular discourse, Australians—non-Aboriginal and Aboriginal—learn about Aboriginal people through their medical behaviors and illnesses. Before developing this argument further, it is necessary to examine how Aboriginal people living in a remote community conceptualize and experience ill health.

Yapa and Kardiya

Lying on the northern edge of the Tanami Desert, Lajamanu was established in 1949 to settle the formerly nomadic Warlpiri people.[4] Originally named Hooker Creek, the community's location was chosen primarily for its distance from white towns and proximity to pastoral leases, where Warlpiri people were expected to work for rations. Consequently, the settlement was placed well north of the region traditionally inhabited by Warlpiri people.[5] Relating the story of his family's arrival in Hooker Creek, one elderly man said, "We really didn't want to come. We said we didn't know that place, not proper way. But they sent us anyway. Now look at all the children. They play in the streets, like they belong here. They don't know that this is not their home, not really." The older residents of Lajamanu recall that the early years of the community were often characterized by hardship and food shortages. The first nurse to visit Hooker Creek, Ellen Kettle (1991, 1.311), described the settlement as "desolate, drought ridden and populated with sick and hungry people." By 1960, over two-thirds of the Warlpiri population was settled in communities supervised by the government (Meggitt 1962, 29).

Approximately 600 kilometers from the town of Katherine, Lajamanu was, and continues to be, one of the most remote communities in

Australia. The non-Aboriginal workers that temporarily resided in the settlement during the 1970s and 1980s dubbed it "Little Siberia." In spite of its remoteness, Lajamanu is the second most populous Warlpiri community and home to about 700 inhabitants. It has a small shop, service station, school, police station, and clinic to meet the needs of its people. In many ways, Lajamanu is typical of other remote Aboriginal communities in the Northern Territory. Many children do not finish school. Unemployment is widespread, leading many to depend on welfare payments provided by the government. Food purchased from the local shop is expensive and few people are adequately nourished. Most homes are in need of repair: Stopped drains, clogged toilets, broken stoves, and damaged locks are common. Resources, food, and living quarters are routinely shared with family and friends.

When I first arrived in 1996 my initial research proposal sought to understand how the clinic and biomedical care were socially situated within the community. I intended to focus primarily on clinic utilization. Although I had an interest in exploring the activities of Warlpiri healers, I was concerned this could be a sensitive subject that people would not wish to discuss with a non-Indigenous anthropologist. After presenting my research proposal to the Lajamanu community council for approval, I was told that the clinic was not an appropriate location to study healing. One man described it as "rubbish," while another said it did not help people at all. Instead of basing my research in the clinic, the council stressed that I was to learn "*yapa* [Aboriginal] way." I was told that I would only be allowed to interview non-Aboriginal medical professionals after first spending an extended period of time learning from Warlpiri people. I agreed. Revising my project, I moved to Lajamanu and conducted twenty-six months of fieldwork. My initial concerns about gaining access to Warlpiri healing knowledge proved unfounded. After several months, I began additional research in the clinic, where medical staff were eager to share their perspectives. I forged social ties with Aboriginal residents as an adopted family member, and with non-Aboriginal health professionals as a colleague. I have repeatedly returned to Lajamanu since my initial fieldwork ended, maintaining relationships and conducting additional research.

As I discovered in my first meeting with the council, Warlpiri people made a clear distinction between Aboriginal ways of being and non-Aboriginal ones. In Lajamanu, as in the rest of the Northern Territory, the social world of Aboriginal people is structured by race (Cowlishaw 2001;

Trigger 1992). Two of the first Warlpiri words that I learned were *yapa* (Aboriginal people) and *kardiya* (white people). These words were not only used by the Warlpiri to denote individuals; they formed a system of classification that was applied to many aspects of the material and social world. *Yapa-kurlangu* (belonging to Aboriginal people) included activities such as hunting, gathering, speaking Warlpiri, attending ceremony, obeying gender norms, and engaging in demand sharing. Indicating beliefs and practices that were regarded as traditional and existing prior to contact, *yapa-kurlangu* embodied Aboriginality. In contrast, *kardiya-kurlangu* (belonging to white people) denoted epistemologies, materials, and expertise that were introduced as a result of the non-Aboriginal settlement of Australia and included commercial foods, bank accounts, English, and saying "please" or "thank you." Illnesses and treatments were also conceptualized in terms of this division. Referring to the clinic, one man said, "All of that medicine; that is *kardiya-kurlangu*."

Lajamanu residents suffered from a variety of diseases and the *kardiya-kurlangu* clinic was a popular source of treatment. The clinic logbook records that over a six-month period an average of forty-seven people a day presented for treatment. On what nurses referred to as a light day between thirty and forty people would come to the clinic for treatment, whereas a heavy day could entail as few as two or three nurses examining upwards of eighty people in fewer than seven hours. Clinic services, including examinations, lab tests, and medications, were provided free of charge. While money was available for a resident doctor, staffing difficulties could lead to the position remaining vacant for months. When this occurred, the community relied on regular but short visits from doctors in Katherine. Funds were also available for Aboriginal Health Workers, but qualified individuals often chose not to work for extended periods at the clinic. The Lajamanu Community Health Centre was consequently primarily staffed by nurses as were many remote area clinics. Most were female and all were non-Aboriginal.[6]

Nurses comprise 36 percent of the workforce of the Northern Territory Department of Health and Families and play the largest role in clinical diagnosis and treatment in the bush (Northern Territory Department of Health 2007, 117). While many nurses are employed in Darwin or Alice Springs, others choose to staff remote area clinics, often the sole location of clinical care in Aboriginal settlements. Due to a shortage of doctors and medical specialists, nurses working in remote clinics must deal with a range of medical activities, usually covered by a variety of health care professionals in an urban setting. These include dispensing drugs, performing administrative tasks, coordinating visits for allied health professionals and physicians, as well as treating a steady stream of patients (Cramer 2005; Kennedy 1997). In Lajamanu, nurses reported that bandaging minor cuts and injuries, treating infectious diseases, managing chronic illness, giving injections, performing prenatal checkups, and distributing pharmaceutical drugs occupied most of their day. Patients suffering from severe conditions such as heart attacks, strokes, severed arteries, and broken skulls were evacuated by air to Katherine Hospital for more comprehensive care.

When I began fieldwork in 1996 the Lajamanu Community Health Centre, as with most remote care facilities, was managed by the Territory Health Services, a branch of the Northern Territory Government. The following year, the Northern Territory and Commonwealth governments began the Katherine West Coordinated Care Trial, aimed at improving chronic disease treatment and increasing Aboriginal participation in health service management. In an effort to encourage self-determination, the Territory Health Services ceded management of the clinic to the Katherine West Health Board, an Aboriginal-led organization. Although the trial has since ended, the change in management became permanent. The Lajamanu clinic is now one of a growing number of community controlled health centers in the Northern Territory. Despite being officially administered by Aboriginal people, the clinic continues to be considered a *kardiya-kurlangu* space.

In addition to *kardiya-kurlangu* facilities and technologies, Warlpiri people also used *yapa-kurlangu* therapies, such as bush medicines and *yawalyu*. Bush medicines, comprised mainly of plant materials or animal fat, were used to heal a variety of complaints, such as coughs, wounds, and sores.[7] Every adult, and many children, have some knowledge of bush medicines. Most substances are either rubbed directly on the skin or inhaled, usually after being boiled in water. Less than 10 percent of medicinal plants are taken internally, unlike biomedical healing aids (Latz 1995, 61). Bush medicines were more highly praised when compared to pharmaceuticals. I was often told that bush medicines were one of the most effective ways of treating a cold. After receiving a severe burn on his leg, James, 16 years old, commented that the best form of treatment was *yapa* way—placing mud on the injury. He added that bandages obtained at the clinic blocked the flow of air around the wound and prevented it from healing properly. Despite the assertions of many Warlpiri people, very few used bush remedies on a regular basis. James made his statement with a large dressing on his leg that he received at the clinic. Regardless of the overwhelming endorsement of the efficacy of *yapa* healing aids, including bush medicines, they are employed far less than pharmaceuticals, which are easier to obtain. However, lack of use does not imply that Warlpiri people doubt the effectiveness of bush medicines. Women also possessed their own healing rituals, *yawalyu*, which could be performed to treat specific symptoms, such as swelling, soreness, pain or a fever, as well as to promote the entire well-being of the community. These songs often focused on personal, procreative, and pediatric health.

Each of these therapies—whether *yapa-kurlangu* or *kardiya-kurlangu*—are only considered to be effective in treating "physical" illness. The result of accidents, viruses, cold weather, genetics, and high blood sugar, physical illnesses are thought to exclusively afflict the corporeal body. In contrast, "spiritual" illnesses are believed to also afflict the soul and are classified as *yapa-kurlangu*. Biomedical practitioners and technologies are viewed as unable to diagnose or treat spiritual illness. As one man commented, "Those nurses don't know everything. We have *yapa* sickness that they can't see." Spiritual illness can be caused by being ensorcelled, breaking customary laws such as treading on sacred land, or seeing a restricted object. Ghosts and human sorcerers are most commonly accused of sending spiritual illness by magically inserting a small piece of sharpened bone into the victim's body. Symptoms of spiritual illness can include fever, chills, vomiting, and achiness, but the only way to obtain a diagnosis and treatment is to consult a *ngangkari*—Aboriginal healer. Visiting a *ngangkari* is a common occurrence that can take place almost anywhere and at anytime—in homes, at football matches, or card games. During a typical consultation the *ngangkari* places his hands on the patient's body, transferring a magical substance that locates any implanted bones and removes them. James said, "You gotta get out that bone. Nothing else, no needle, no pills, will make you better." In Lajamanu, suffering from spiritual illness and consulting *ngangkari* was not uncommon. Sorcery, ghosts, and *ngangkari* were as much a part of everyday life as diabetes and clinical treatment. Nevertheless, a clear distinction has been made between these two realms of healing. Jessica noted, "You *kardiya* have doctors, but we *yapa* have *ngangkari*."

Warlpiri narratives about illness tend to present dichotomous categories and treatment guidelines: *ngangkari* can only treat spiritual illness and medical staff can only treat physical illness. Although statements entrenching the division between *yapa-kurlangu* and *kardiya-kurlangu*—between Aboriginality and whiteness—pervade health conversations in Lajamanu, individuals seeking treatment for an actual illness seldom restricted their choice of therapy. Despite assertions regarding the incommensurability of Aboriginal and non-Aboriginal practices, Warlpiri people have little trouble moving back and forth between *yapa-kurlangu* and *kardiya-kurlangu*. In many instances, people concurrently employed both therapies to treat a single illness episode. Taking antibiotics while seeing a *ngangkari* was not unusual. But despite the use of multiple treatment regimes, individuals regularly credited *yapa* remedies rather than *kardiya* ones. When discussing the efficacy of various treatments, Betty recounted a recent episode in which doctors referred her to a hospital in Adelaide to undergo an operation for a "bad heart." Regardless of the medical diagnosis, Betty sensed that her illness was not physical. She said, "Those *kardiya* doctors, they couldn't see really." Following the surgery, Betty had three bones magically removed from her heart. She was adamant that if she had not received this spiritual treatment, she would have died. The operation, Betty added, didn't help her at all.

Given the context of everyday life, it seems logical that Aboriginal people would—and do—use a variety of technologies and tactics. The social world of Aboriginal people is far more complex and integrated than dichotomous models indicate. Nevertheless, narratives of incommensurabilities and chasms remain because they strategically construct and maintain notions of Aboriginality. While parallel treatment was the norm, the notional division between *yapa* and *kardiya* was so habitual that I never heard anyone credit the simultaneous use of therapies. Yet, concurrent treatment illustrates the pervasive slippage between the way social relations are represented and the way that they are lived. There is an imperative across Australia to evoke racial difference despite the reality of integration (Sullivan 2006, 255). Contrasting assumptions of divergence with the everyday realities experienced by Aboriginal people in Katherine, Merlan (2005, 169) urges an examination of "the 'inter-' of categories, understandings, modes of practical action, as reproduced and reshaped in interaction, interrelationship and event—sometimes in engagement with whites—rather than pre-given." This task can be accomplished by shifting the focus from idealized treatment models to actual behaviors. In this way, medicine ceases to be a realm of confusion and becomes the product of ongoing interactions. Rather than reducing Aboriginal ill health to cultural misunderstandings, cultural loss, or the pathology of culture, I intend to situate disease within a framework of experience, sociality, and resistance. It is to these themes that I will now turn.

Experience, Sociality, and Resistance

In recent years anthropology has given greater attention to experience and sensation, acknowledging that illness is felt and lived (Csordas 1990; Good 1994; Jackson 1996; Kleinman and Kleinman 1996). While ideas of race and difference structure medical dialogue, the residents of Lajamanu also inhabit a world of physical discomfort and chronic disease. Consequently, understanding illness requires an understanding of this experience. Martin's earlier statement that he was not suffering from illness despite being a diabetic is telling. In Lajamanu, the ubiquity of suffering—physical and social—is taken for granted. Frequent bouts of disease are not always viewed as symptomatic of a larger problem. Warlpiri people are accustomed to repeated episodes of ill health. While health professionals worry over high morbidity rates, many Warlpiri people continue to go about their lives believing that they are in good health. Over half of the Aboriginal people living in the Northern Territory self-assessed their health as "excellent/very good," despite enduring the worst health in the nation (Australian Bureau of Statistics 2006, table 19).[8] For many Warlpiri people—including Martin and Catherine—*being* sick is contingent on *feeling* sick. The everyday sensations of Lajamanu's residents—headaches, dizziness, hunger, and obesity—transform symptoms of illness into conditions of life. Lewis (1993, 206) asserts that where disease and hardship are prevalent, individuals "are used to putting up with the flies, the scabs, and the pain; they have different expectations, a different level of tolerance." As a result of not feeling ill, many individuals suffering from chronic illness choose not to take medication. Martin, like other diabetics, admitted that he *knows* he will always suffer from the disease. But because he does not *feel* sick, Martin sees no reason to monitor his blood sugar or take pharmaceuticals.

Illness experience and care seeking are lifelong processes. While affecting the individual, disease also impacts the community. Stories of sickness circulate at the shop, at evening card games, and during phone calls to friends and relatives. While ostensibly concerned with diagnoses, these conversations can also hypothesize transgressions, comment upon moral character, and express political viewpoints. Tales of sorcery or cancer can highlight disagreements between families, age groups, and genders. In addition to discussing symptoms, community residents provide care for one another, solicited through demands for special foods, hot tea, non-prescription pharmaceuticals, bush medicines, or other healing aids. The process of looking after sick individuals is firmly embedded in notions of relatedness and sociality (Dussart 2010). Individuals will choose a *ngang-kari* based upon social relationships, often preferring a close family member. Likewise, consultations with doctors, nurses, and Aboriginal Health Workers are also social. If possible, individuals will select medical professionals with whom they are personally familiar or related. Similar demands are also made of medical professionals. Patients can insist on being given prescription pharmaceuticals or after-hours care. Consequently, illness becomes a nexus around which personhood is expressed and relationships are maintained. Through sickness—attending the clinic, taking pills, maintaining special diets—Warlpiri sociality—selfhood, autonomy, kin relations, gender norms, and reciprocity—is enacted.

Illness narratives and behaviors reflect a range of relationships, including those among Aboriginal people, non-Aboriginal people, and the state. While the actual choices that individuals make to treat their sicknesses are often ignored or deviate from the notional division between *yapa* and *kardiya*, this dichotomy did reflect a reality of a different sort. Whereas many Warlpiri people were unemployed, the approximately forty non-Aboriginal people living in Lajamanu were there expressly to work, supplying services and expertise. Schoolteachers, shop managers, electricians, carpenters, case managers, police officers, nurses, doctors, outstation resource personnel, mechanics, and accountants were all non-Aboriginal. While Warlpiri individuals called Lajamanu home, non-Aboriginal residents saw themselves as temporary workers. They seldom stayed in the community for more than a couple of years. Some left after only a few weeks. Non-Aboriginal employees in Aboriginal communities not only manage services and provide skilled labor; they are "part of a systematic relationship between the nation and Indigenous people" (Cowlishaw 2010, 57). In Lajamanu, daily life—residing in a home, receiving income, purchasing food, and sharing a meal with friends—informed and reinforced racial difference.

Each non-Aboriginal family was allotted a single home for their stay in Lajamanu. Aside from a row of flats at the rear of the clinic, homes reserved for non-Aboriginal workers were almost exclusively located in a relatively circumscribed region of the community. Given the high percentage of workers who were young and unmarried, it was common for non-Aboriginal dwellings to accommodate a single resident, which was a stark contrast to overcrowded Warlpiri homes. Aboriginal and non-Aboriginal residents of Lajamanu were also subject to different regulations regarding the consumption of alcohol. In 1979, Lajamanu became a "dry" community—the possession of alcohol was prohibited within a ten-mile radius of the settlement—and the vehicle of anyone caught illegally bringing alcohol into the community was confiscated by the police. While it was possible for non-Aboriginal workers to apply for a permit allowing them to possess alcohol, few chose to follow this procedure. It was common knowledge that the police would not prosecute fellow non-Aboriginal people for this offense. Non-Aboriginal people would often sit outside drinking beer while Warlpiri residents walked by, conscious of the heavy penalties Aboriginal people faced if they attempted to bring alcohol into the community.

Despite living together in a small community, there was little social contact between Aboriginal and non-Aboriginal people outside the business environment. Many social gatherings, particularly those that took place inside private homes, were segregated.[9] On the weekends or evenings, non-Aboriginal workers would congregate to drink and talk about their lives. I never witnessed an Aboriginal person present at any of these events. Similarly, Aboriginal people seldom invited non-Aboriginal workers to share meals, attend ceremonies, or participate in card games. A popular topic of conversation at these get-togethers was race. Warlpiri people complained that *kardiya* were racist, had little respect for Aboriginal people, and were given preferential treatment. I was told, for instance that the Northern Territory government built new homes for non-Aboriginal workers, while only painting the exterior walls of Warlpiri houses. In contrast, non-Aboriginal workers complained that Warlpiri people were lazy, irresponsible, and incapable of looking after themselves. At one non-Aboriginal social gathering a schoolteacher asked, "What would they do if we weren't here? I bet this place would fall apart."

Attitudes and perceptions of racial difference were entrenched, pervasive, and performed as a routine part of life. Assertions of Aboriginal irresponsibility suffused non-Aboriginal narratives surrounding health and illness, which in turn were tied to disputes regarding the value of Aboriginality. Race not only structured relations between people, it was also a tool through which identity was managed. For instance, some nurses commented that Aboriginal people were irresponsible and did not look after their own health or that of their children. A persistent topic of conversation among nursing staff was the high rates of pharmaceutical noncompliance and late presentation. When distributed, pills were often not taken according to the required dosage or frequency. More commonly, individuals did not collect their medication at all. On a monthly basis, the clinic disposed of hundreds of pharmaceuticals that were not picked up by Aboriginal patients. In addition to complaints of noncompliance, Warlpiri people were also criticized for unnecessarily consulting the clinic after hours, often waking the on call nurse in the middle of the night. During clinical consultations, non-Aboriginal medical staff regularly admonished Warlpiri people for their poor health behavior. Complaining about the high rate of noncompliance, one nurse said, "It's their own fault they are dying."

For Lajamanu's Aboriginal residents, health and medical care were also idioms through which a larger struggle of signification and, ultimately, resistance was being waged. Playing a major role in the social life of the community, the clinic and its staff were the subject of many conversations. The vast majority of people seemed to agree that the clinic provided a much needed service. Nevertheless, the clinic was also a target for criticism and dissatisfaction. Residents complained about its personnel and services, often stating that nurses were incompetent and racist. Robert added that although the clinic claimed to be concerned with health, he believed it was an institution through which *kardiya* controlled *yapa*. Despite being community controlled through the oversight of the Katherine West Health Board, the clinic continues to be considered an embodiment of whiteness. Comparing the community controlled clinic to the period when Aboriginal people were wards of the state, Robert said, "It is still like the old days, only newer, different." Robert, like many others who complained about the clinic and its staff, seldom confronted the nurses directly. Most negative comments were shared outside the clinic. In some cases, however, dissatisfaction and anger over the actions of medical personnel led to quarrels and confrontations between nurses and patients. Referring to the nursing staff, one woman said, "You have to be firm. Tell them to fuck off sometimes." Many residents could recount tales of cursing at nurses. During my research in the clinic, I witnessed a number of altercations that ended in harsh words. Infrequently, these conflicts could result in vandalism and assault. In one instance, a nurse took refuge at the police station claiming that Aboriginal people were threatening her life.

While notions of Indigeneity might have been borne out of a history of colonialism, medical knowledge, and government interventions, non-Indigenous people are not in complete control of these meanings. Although constrained by existing constructions of Aboriginality, these conceptualizations are nevertheless a site of contestation. *Ampe Akelyernemane Meke Mekarle "Little Children Are Sacred"* reports that Aboriginal informants stated that child sexual abuse was rare prior to the non-Indigenous settlement of Australia. Furthermore, the current levels of abuse were thought to be the result of "the erosion of traditional restraints and behavior that has been 'learnt' from the treatment received at the hands of the colonisers" (Board of Inquiry into the Protection of Aboriginal Children from Sexual Abuse 2007, 139). In these Aboriginal narratives, blame for child abuse is leveled at colonization and non-Indigenous interference in Indigenous lives. Aboriginal people are particularly able to engage with dominant ideas of race through everyday interactions with non-Aboriginal people (Cowlishaw 2004). One arena in which this occurs is clinical interaction and medical narratives. Health and illness have become vehicles through which Aboriginal people are able to address the history of colonialism as well as contemporary political conditions. Disease and suffering are markers of identity that embody relations between Indigenous and non-Indigenous Australians.

For Indigenous people, medicine provides a commentary on race relations through discussions of etiology and efficacy: *Yapa-kurlangu* remedies, such as bush medicines, are valued more highly than pharmaceuticals; white nurses are said to be unable to treat *yapa* disease; tales of biomedical treatment highlight clashes between suffering Aboriginal people and racist non-Aboriginal medical professionals. Disease, pathology and biomedical treatment are repeatedly linked to a history of colonization and government interference, whereas life prior to contact is equated with vitality. Integrating medical discourse with local categories of race, Warlpiri notions of diagnoses and treatments are able to comment critically upon the meaning and value of Aboriginality. Similar dynamics have been noted elsewhere. Examining Indigenous medical narratives in Bolivia, Crandon-Malamud (1997, 87) writes, "In an environment that is . . . medically pluralistic, people draw on multiple medical ideologies. As they do so, their medical dialogue reflects, involves, and contributes to the construction of political, economic, ideological, and social relations. Through medical dialogue, ethnic groups negotiate the meaning of ethnic identity and affiliation, and therefore ethnic relations." Warlpiri statements utilize medicine as a competitive field on which dominant racial metaphors can be contested. While non-Aboriginal Australians employ health disparities to demonstrate Aboriginal inaction and the need for government supervision, Warlpiri dialogues of disease invert these meanings.

In Aboriginal communities, where the repetition and dramatization of stories and encounters is an important aspect of everyday life (Sansom, 1980), medical narratives are a form of social action. Through the enactment of health, disease, and treatment, ethnicity is performed in social situations where actors are conscious of intent and audience. Daily interactions in Aboriginal communities are one way in which individuals position themselves and others within a social world. Obtaining treatment from non-Aboriginal nurses at the clinic presents an opportunity for Warlpiri people to engage with dominant notions of Aboriginality. Shaped by popular narratives regarding Aboriginal behavior, the forms of expression available to Warlpiri people are limited. Cursing at nurses, throwing away medication, and failing to appear for appointments are a few of the ways in which residents demonstrate difference and defiance. As a result, performing Aboriginality to non-Aboriginal people often entails enacting the predominant stereotypes, thereby reaffirming the line between white and black.

Enduring Afflictions

Through a focus on disease and medicine, this book seeks to shift understandings of Aboriginal action from popular notions of cultural exceptionalism—which is often invoked in postcolonial and neoliberal perspectives—to those of everyday experience and contemporary sociality. Rather than reifying tradition or casting it as inflexible or incommensurable with modernity, I will illustrate the ways in which Aboriginal lives are integrated and complex. In Lajamanu, biomedicine has been incorporated into Warlpiri cosmological beliefs and customary regulations, and, as a result, is utilized as any other local institution. Illness is an idiom through which social relations are mobilized and contested. Governments have used medicine to construct notions of Indigeneity and, likewise, Indigenous people also deploy medical discourse to critically comment upon race relations. Rather than a source for misunderstanding and disjuncture, medicine can be conceived of as a communication channel through which Aboriginal and non-Aboriginal people speak to one another.

Examining the opening of a bridge in Zululand, Gluckman (1940) scrutinized the interactions of the participants to challenge assumptions that Zulu beliefs were at odds with English ones. This book similarly provides an ethnography of relationships, but instead of a bridge, my focus will be on illness narratives, diagnosis, and treatment. Like Gluckman, I will not only explore the beliefs of Indigenous people, but will discuss those of white Australians as well. While anthropologists have examined Aboriginal reactions to government policy and interventions, there has been little systematic recording or analysis of the everyday interactions between Aboriginal and non-Aboriginal people (Cowlishaw 2010, 52). This book seeks to redress this imbalance by demonstrating that, for all of the concern about miscomprehension and incommensurability between Aboriginal and non-Aboriginal people and ways of life, people generally understand each other all too well.

Recounting the everyday lives of individuals—Aboriginal and non-Aboriginal—living in Lajamanu, I demonstrate that their concerns, tactics, and strategies are born out of, and represent, the contemporary social, economic, and embodied contexts of remote Aboriginal communities. I argue that while social norms and propensities impact Aboriginal action in Lajamanu, these are, in part, derived from the experience of poverty, constant illness, and structural violence. Drawing on research conducted in a Boston homeless shelter, Desjarlais (1996, 1997) examines the way in which the practice of daily life fundamentally alters perception. In the shelter, lives are structured by negotiating public spaces, bumming cigarettes, holding onto words, pacing, and watching television. Desjarlais states that daily life is best characterized as "struggling along." He writes, "To 'struggle along' was to proceed with great difficulty while trying at times to do away with or avoid the constraints and hazards strewn in one's path. The struggles implied strenuous efforts against opposition, hitting up against a world filled with noise, voices, bodies, pains, distractions, poverty, displacements, and bureaucratic powers" (1997, 19). The process of struggling along—dealing with the concerns and hardships of everyday life—influenced the way in which residents of the homeless shelter perceived the world and acted within it.

In some respects, a similar situation exists in Lajamanu. Structural violence and social suffering have become part of the everyday lives of Aboriginal people in remote Australia (Austin-Broos 2009, 9).[10]

Warlpiri negotiate a world of dust, poverty, spirit beings, social responsibilities, and government services. The social and material conditions in Indigenous communities—high rates of disease, few functioning facilities, low income, unemployment, and reliance on services provided by non-Indigenous workers—influence how people respond to the world around them. Drawing inspiration from Desjarlais, I believe the phrase best able to encapsulate daily lives in remote Aboriginal communities is "enduring afflictions." On one hand, illness itself is lasting. High rates of mortality and morbidity are not declining and chronic disease is particularly prevalent. Skin sores, hunger, obesity, headaches, and bodily discomfort are a continual feature of existence. But illness is not only enduring, it is also endured. Aboriginal people routinely bear these conditions. Illness and dis-ease are integrated into daily life. To endure affliction, however, does not entail remaining passive. Aboriginal people are able to engage and contest dominant paradigms and government interventions through illness, medical narratives, and health behaviors. The very act of enduring—of being sick and accepting illness as normative—is an assertion of power and agency.

Focusing on the ways in which illness is experienced and interpreted in Lajamanu, each of the following chapters explores the interplay of meanings, constraints, possibilities, and tactics. Chapter 2 examines the way in which notions of Indigeneity and whiteness are created and entrenched through narratives of chronic illness and food. Chronic conditions such as diabetes disproportionately affect Indigenous peoples around the globe. These high rates are often linked to changes in food consumption. Consequently, to get to grips with the reality of chronic illness it is necessary to understand food as a symbol and a commodity. In Australia, the distribution of rations such white flour, tea, sugar, and tinned meat to Aboriginal people acted as a strategy of settlement and assimilation as well as an idiom through which knowledge of Aboriginal people could be constructed. Today, food continues to structure social relations. On one hand, food consumption is impacted by norms of reciprocity and a reliance on welfare payments. On the other, stressing that medical researchers have proved bush foods are superior to commercial ones, Warlpiri people utilize the language of science, medicine, and nutrition to demonstrate the pathology of white control and the vitality of Aboriginality. Aboriginal people engage with economic, social, and political circumstances through food narratives and the act of eating.

The third chapter focuses on beliefs often characterized as traditional to demonstrate that Indigenous cosmologies, while drawing from the past, also reflect recent debates over the value and sustainability of Indigeneity. I situate Warlpiri concepts—including the soul, ancestral beings, and local healers—within the everyday environment of biomedical treatment, government intervention, and racial difference. Consequently, so-called traditional beliefs are firmly embedded in experiences of affliction and marginalization. While these narratives are inherently social, highlighting personal disputes and transgressions, I argue that explanations garnered from non-Aboriginal cosmologies can fulfill a similar role. Using ethnographic examples, I demonstrate that biomedical accounts can be employed in much the same way as sorcery accusations, acting as a medium through which tensions within the community are voiced. National and international narratives of genetics, chronic illness, and UFOs are made local, creating accounts through which Warlpiri people socially situate themselves and others.

Given the continuing existence of local medical beliefs and practices, there has been a tendency to cast Indigenous people as having a choice between two conflicting medical systems: biomedical and Indigenous. Some health researchers and medical professionals view the existence of Indigenous beliefs as discouraging clinical care and assert that diagnoses are the foremost factor influencing illness behavior. Challenging this assumption, Chapter 4 charts the way in which one man concurrently employed a range of diagnoses and therapies during an extended illness episode. In actuality, *ngangkari* and nurses were treated similarly: with protocols that might or might not be the most comfortable, accessible, socially acceptable, or expedient way to end disease. Rather than realistic guides for action that reflect the reality of illness behavior, statements stressing the separation of medical systems function as modalities through which social relations are articulated and notions of racial difference are reinforced. Consequently, crediting a *ngangkari* after receiving clinical treatment is not the result of biological ignorance, but rather a meaningful articulation of the value of Aboriginality.

Chapter 5 examines interactions and narratives surrounding the distribution and use of pharmaceuticals. Despite having free access to prescription medication, each month hundreds of pills were discarded in Lajamanu. I argue that prescription pharmaceuticals not only treat illness, they also act as a physical locus around which relationships between

Indigenous and non-Indigenous people are enacted. Although barriers to taking pharmaceuticals include misunderstandings, lack of storage facilities, overprescribing, frequent medication changes, and a lack of noticeable symptoms, these features were seldom discussed in Lajamanu. Instead, nursing staff complained that noncompliance was the result of Aboriginal irresponsibility and laziness. In contrast, Aboriginal patients accused medical staff of racism and incompetence, claiming that pharmaceuticals were unnecessary or harmful. Narratives of noncompliance constituted a public forum through which whiteness and Aboriginality were performed and negotiated through entrenched, habitual, and constitutive racial rhetoric.

Chapter 6 asks the question: What is Indigenous empowerment? Through an investigation of initiatives that incorporate Indigenous medical professionals and management into the clinical care system of the Northern Territory, I argue that the government's notion of Indigenous empowerment is very different from that of Warlpiri people. Despite the introduction of the Aboriginal Health Worker Program and Aboriginal control of local medical facilities, Lajamanu residents complain that little has changed in day-to-day life of the clinic. Interactions between nurses and patients remain hostile, Aboriginal Health Workers refuse employment, and medical services are limited. I assert that policies of empowerment essentialize ethnic categories, underestimate the omnipresence of government in Australia's rural regions, and overestimate the interest of Aboriginal people in taking over health care services. Examining Warlpiri political structures, I conclude that Aboriginal people prefer to allow non-Aboriginal people to embody responsibility. Consequently, Aboriginal reluctance to take over health services can be viewed as a form of Indigenous action.

Chapter 7 brings the book full circle with an examination of what is commonly referred to as the gap in health between Indigenous and non-Indigenous Australians. Often assumed to be self-evident and empirical, health statistics embed the difference between Aboriginal and non-Aboriginal people while being marshaled to argue for government intervention. In an effort to reduce high rates of morbidity and mortality, government and health advocates have endorsed a number of programs and policies. I explore four themes that can be found throughout many initiatives focusing on Indigenous populations: improving essential services and community infrastructure; developing education programs for Indigenous people; improving health services through primary health care; and educating non-Indigenous health professionals in a cross-cultural approach. Weaving together threads from previous chapters, I examine how the constraints of life in remote Aboriginal communities—poverty, norms, knowledge, and experience—impact these goals. In doing so, I demonstrate the ways in which anthropological understandings can be used to assess health policy pragmatically and offer lessons for future initiatives.

After researching Aboriginal health for over fifteen years, I am still struck by the difference between the rhetoric and the reality. On one hand, narratives, stories, statistics, opinions, and promises all seem to focus on a gap, a fundamental difference between Aboriginal and non-Aboriginal people. I have heard nurses speculate why "they don't take better care of themselves." I have read books and health policies that attribute continuing poor health to biomedicine's ill fit within the cultural context of Aboriginal communities. Parallel to these narratives, run the everyday lives of Lajamanu residents, which are far more complex. Aboriginal people navigate a world of government interventions, poverty, and illness that is embedded in a social environment of racial difference, behavioral norms, and practical strategies. People make due and get by. For the residents of Lajamanu, illness is simultaneously a mode of social expression, a political tactic, and a personal experience.

CHAPTER 2

Food, Meaning, and Economy

Worldwide, Indigenous people are disproportionately affected by chronic illnesses such as diabetes mellitus, hypertension, cardiovascular disease, and renal failure. For Indigenous communities, these ailments are relatively new. It was not until the mid-twentieth century that epidemiological research began documenting a steep rise in rates of chronic disease (Ferreira and Lang 2006, 11). These trends are certainly visible in Australia's Northern Territory. Since 1977, Aboriginal deaths from non-communicable chronic lifestyle diseases have been steadily increasing (Thomas et al. 2006). It is estimated that 11.5 percent of Aboriginal Territorians suffer from hypertension, while 13.4 percent have type 2 diabetes (Zhao et al. 2008). Almost 60 percent of the Aboriginal population in the Northern Territory will have at least one chronic condition between the ages of thirty-five and forty-four which will require continual medical treatment, often with multiple drugs, for the rest of their lives (Hoy et al. 2007, 181). Research suggests that 77 percent of the life expectancy difference between Aboriginal and non-Aboriginal Territorians is the result of these illnesses (Zhao and Dempsey 2006).

In many instances, rising rates of chronic illness are linked to changes in food consumption. After their settlement on reservations and reserves, many Indigenous diets shifted from hunted and gathered foods to processed commercial ones. In the Northern Territory, refined carbohydrates have comprised a disproportionate amount of food intake for at least the last two decades. Four items—table sugar (16 percent), flour (13 percent), bread (11 percent), and milk powder (8 percent)—provide approximately half of an individual's total energy intake (Brimblecombe and O'Dea 2009, 550). Fat ingestion has been recorded as twice that of non-Aboriginal Australians and salt intake as over five times the recommended amount (Northern Territory Department of Health 1995b, 5). Forty-five percent of fat intake has been attributed to the consumption of fatty meats while sixty percent of sugar intake is derived from white sugar, amounting to approximately thirty-eight teaspoons per person per day (Harrison 1991, 127). Meanwhile, the consumption of nutritious food items is minimal, particularly in remote communities.

On a daily basis, 20.7 percent of Aboriginal people living in remote regions do not eat vegetables as compared to only 1 percent of the non-remote Aboriginal population (Australian Bureau of Statistics 2006, table 22). Overall, fruit and vegetables provide only 1 percent and 5 percent (respectively) of daily calories (Brimblecombe and O'Dea 2009, 550). The result of chronically poor diets, Aboriginal communities in the Northern Territory have significantly higher rates of obesity and malnutrition (Russell et al. 2004). In 1994, about 29 percent of the Aboriginal population in the Katherine region were overweight, while 17 percent were obese, and the remaining 15 percent were underweight (Aboriginal and Torres Strait Islander Commission 1994, 23). Since that time, the incidence of obesity in the Northern Territory has risen to 20 percent (Australian Bureau of Statistics 2006, table 21) but has been recorded as high as 38 percent in some Aboriginal communities (Hoy et al. 2007). Inadequate nutrition contributes to over 16 percent of the burden of disease nationally, but in the Northern Territory this number is even higher (Lee et al. 2009, 547).

Lajamanu epitomizes many of these statistics. Diabetes affects a significant portion of the population with some cases diagnosed in residents as young as fifteen years old. Large quantities of white flour and sugar are purchased from the shop, while fatty foods obtained from the takeaway are a regular staple of midday meals. Fresh fruits and vegetables are seldom eaten. While a number of health campaigns have attempted to foster nutritional awareness, eating habits have not changed significantly in the last decade. Nevertheless, Aboriginal residents are well aware of the dangers of consuming foods high in fat and sugar. I often witnessed Warlpiri people complaining about the poor nutritional quality of food served by the local takeaway only to find them purchasing lunch there later the same day. Although many community residents vowed to hunt and gather as a healthy alternative to commercial food, very few regularly ate bush foods. Statistical data illustrate a variety of the factors influencing chronic disease rates, but this information alone is unable to give meaning to the daily events and actions that structure Aboriginal lives.

Through food narratives and consumption, Aboriginal people engage with everyday economic, social, and political realities. To better illuminate the complex representations and choices surrounding food in Lajamanu, it is necessary to examine food as both a commodity and a symbol. On one hand, food is an article of trade. In remote Aboriginal communities, food prices are significantly higher than in urban centers, while incomes are significantly lower. A reliance on government welfare payments often limits when and what kinds of food can be purchased. But food is not only bought and sold, it is also exchanged. An ethos of reciprocity pervades Aboriginal communities, where cash is used to reproduce social relations (Peterson 1993). As Heil (2006, 103) notes, "It is part of a system that constitutes and reconstitutes sociality by putting particular emphases on the relationships and obligations *between* people. 'Demand sharing' emphasises the working of the communal social network and, correspondingly, does not encourage a system of individuation or the prioritising of personal values and interests." Underpinned by a variety of social and economic strategies, the dynamics of food consumption not only contextualize continuing high rates of chronic illness, they also draw attention to the ways in which government controlled payments, the enactment of sociality, and bodily experience work together to structure daily life.

While shop prices, welfare payments, and norms of reciprocity shape daily strategies, food also acts as a symbol of race relations. From the earliest contact between white settlers and Aboriginal people, the exchange of food has been imbued with signification. Intended as a means of assimilation, rationing introduced many of the foods that Warlpiri people now blame for causing high rates of chronic illness, including white flour, sugar, and beef. Consequently, diseases such as diabetes are often considered to be non-Indigenous (Lang 2006; Roy 2006; Saethre 2005; Tom-Orme 1993). As with other illness narratives, those surrounding nutrition construct and resist historic and contemporary social relations. Food, nutrition, and chronic disease have become idioms through which colonialism, race, and ethnicity are parleyed. Suffering from diabetes presents Indigenous people with a tool to reconfigure and contest notions of Indigeneity and whiteness.

Rations to Welfare

The way in which food is consumed and conceptualized in Aboriginal communities today is the result of a history of food exchanges in Central

Australia. The availability of food and water has historically structured social relations between Aboriginal people in the Northern Territory as well as their interactions with non-Aboriginal explorers and settlers. Prior to contact, the increased rains of the summer months created reliable water sources that allowed nomadic groups to assemble in larger numbers to conduct ceremonies, arrange marriages, and settle disputes. After the rains ceased and hunting and gathering became more difficult, congregations would fracture into smaller units. Beginning in the late nineteenth century, this pattern was disrupted as Europeans explored and settled the central regions of the continent. Non-Aboriginal people used and depleted water sources relied upon by local Aboriginal groups. Giles (1889, 212) writes, "No doubt these . . . [Aborigines] were dreadfully annoyed to find their little reservoirs discovered by such water-swallowing wretches as they doubtless thought white men and horses to be." During his crossing of the desert in 1896 and 1897 Carnegie (1898) reports capturing a few Aboriginal people, using ropes and later chains as restraints, and attempting to force them to lead him to water.

As pastoralists settled in Central Australia, conflicts over water, land, and cattle predation typified relations between Aboriginal and non-Aboriginal people (Peterson et al. 1978). In an effort to secure their safety and livelihoods, pastoralists sought to introduce a method through which relationships with Aboriginal people could be managed beneficially (Wright 1981, 77-84; May 1994, 40-44). While force and the use of weaponry were common, an alternative strategy was to socially engage Aboriginal people through the distribution of materials, including food. Dried tea leaves, white flour, sugar, and preserved meat were rationed throughout the Northern Territory in towns, missions, and cattle stations. In pursuing a policy of assimilation, the Australian government attempted to use the material and social exchange of rations as a strategy through which white values, manners, and eating habits would be imparted to the Aboriginal population (Rowse 1998). In the process, rations were also seen as a way of encouraging Aboriginal people to sell their labor to cattle stations, thus creating a cheap and much-needed workforce in the bush. It was hoped that through the experiences of employment, queuing up for a ration allotment, and being taught to prepare and consume the distributed food, Aboriginal people would adopt the lifestyle and values of white Australia, including a strong work ethic, timeliness, and hygiene.

Although initially affecting Aboriginal people living in the vicinity of white settlements and pastoral leases, rations came to play a larger role in the remote regions of the Northern Territory over time. During the late nineteenth and early twentieth centuries, Warlpiri people were not dependent upon rations for survival, although settler food was eaten as a supplement to a foraged diet. However, when a severe drought struck Central Australia from 1924 to 1929, the subsequent scarcity of edible plants and animals in the bush necessitated seeking larger amounts of rations from non-Aboriginal people (Meggitt 1962, 24). As towns became an increasingly popular and necessary source of food for Aboriginal people, ration depots were established in the bush. Hoping to prevent additional migration into white settlements, the government encouraged semi-permanent residence around these newly established ration stations. Between 1937 and 1968, ration stations were used to construct a network of Aboriginal communities designed to train Indigenous people for citizenship (Rowse 1998, 147).

The policy of rations for labor was instrumental in the creation of Lajamanu. In 1946 the Tanami region ration depot was moved to Yuendumu, three hundred kilometers northwest of Alice Springs, where four hundred Warlpiri were settled (Meggitt 1962, 29). Since the initial population of Yuendumu consisted of Warlpiri from both the northern and southern Tanami, a new settlement was planned in the north to support the Warlpiri from that region. Hooker Creek, which would later become Lajamanu, was established in 1949 in an effort to encourage Aboriginal labor on cattle stations removed from white urban centers (Peterson et al. 1978).

Meat was to be procured from a herd of bullocks, but due to a lack of rich grazing ground, these cattle took longer to mature. When it became apparent the herd would not be viable for some years, the residents were forced to find other sources of meat, such as the staff's domestic cats (Kettle 1991, 2.73). Although a garden was planted in 1953, the harsh conditions made growing vegetables difficult, particularly enough to supply the entire population. Given the difficulties of producing food locally, the community relied on supplies brought from town (Wild 1975, 17). The journey over bad roads would often result in trucks breaking down, becoming stuck in mud, and eventually arriving after a long hot journey with much of the fresh food spoilt and inedible. Consequently, foods that were easy to transport, would not go rotten, and were inexpensive to buy, were ideal. Flour, sugar, tea leaves, and tinned meat met these criteria and were staple foods of the community. Due to the lack of fresh produce, scurvy was rife for several years to come (Kettle 1991, 2.73).

Although food distribution occurred throughout the Aboriginal settlements of the Northern Territory, the government did not intend rationing to be a permanent strategy. Instead, rationing was viewed as a vital stage in the evolution and eventual assimilation of Aboriginal people into the Australian cash economy. This process would be accomplished, in part, by the gradual introduction of cash wages. Ian Sharp (1966, 162), of the Department of Labor and National Service, wrote that the transition to "equal wages" for Aboriginal pastoral workers would encourage "the handling of cash wages and accepting increasingly the family responsibilities of a normal wage earner." Due to the interference of trade unions, however, the transition to cash wages occurred faster than the government intended. In 1969, rationing abruptly ended. Unemployment payments were initially limited to a minority of the Aboriginal population—those who had either been previously employed or undertaking training. By 1974, unemployment benefits were made universally available to all Aboriginal people. In place of rations, the state had instituted a cash-based regime of government payments to Aboriginal people: welfare. Today, most Aboriginal people living in remote regions of the Northern Territory are not regularly employed and receive the bulk of their income from government assistance payments.

The introduction of universal unemployment benefits was motivated by a marked increase in poverty in Aboriginal communities after 1969. Despite the advent of cash wages, many Aboriginal people did not sell their labor. Previously, communal kitchens would have distributed meals to residents, but now individuals chose to purchase food from local shops. The lack of cash to buy food led to widespread malnutrition. Given the rapid decline in health, administrators and government officials questioned if Aboriginal people could now adequately look after themselves. Rowse (1998, 180) writes, "When cash award wages, training allowances and social service benefits were introduced on settlement in 1969, the 'problem' of the ill-prepared Indigenous family began to appear prolifically in Administration files, under three themes: Were parents willing to look after their families? Did they have the dietary knowledge to do so competently? Could they afford to do so?" In many instances, the answer was "no." In 1970, observers noted that while Aboriginal people purchased food at the local shop or canteen immediately after receiving pay, by the end of the two-week pay cycle, spending was dramatically reduced (Rowse 1998, 238). Lack of food contributed to inadequate child nutrition, which was a particular concern of government officials (Rowse

1998, 180). Today, government apprehension regarding the use of welfare continues. In 2007, the Northern Territory Emergency Response sought to improve child nutrition by placing a significant portion of welfare payments to Aboriginal people in accounts that could only be accessed when purchasing food from local shops.

Although the transition from rations to cash was intended to shift Aboriginal policy from dependency to self-determination, anthropologists have questioned if this move has in fact occurred. In 1977 Robert Paine coined the phrase "welfare colonialism," asserting that government allocations to Indigenous peoples actually entrench social and political dependency. He argues that welfare payments are emblematic of larger incongruities that exist in modern relationships between industrially developed nation states and the Indigenous minorities who inhabit them. On one hand, receiving the dole represents the rights of citizenship; while on the other, the state continues to control economies in Indigenous communities. Peterson (1998; 1999) has argued for a more nuanced approach to welfare colonialism, noting that too often the everyday economic and social realities of welfare are ignored. As he observes, welfare payments allow Aboriginal people to pursue local social and cultural activities, such as playing cards or attending ceremony, without the need to sell their labor in a capitalist market. Thus, cash is used to reproduce and strengthen social relations. This is accomplished, in part, through the redistribution of food purchased at the store.

Rationing and the subsequent introduction of welfare payments not only established a material relationship between Aboriginal and non-Aboriginal people, it also provided a medium through which notions regarding Aboriginality could be created and articulated. The reluctance of Aboriginal people to sell their labor seemed to substantiate labels such as lazy, irresponsible, and dependent. Today one frequently hears non-Aboriginal Australians referring to Aboriginal people as "dole bludgers." Furthermore, labor and health became linked: high rates of chronic lifestyle disease are viewed as a consequence of inadequate nutrition, fostered by a lack of employment. In the way that earlier descriptions of the "Native pox" cast Aboriginal people as morally suspect, so do those of chronic lifestyle diseases. Narratives of social and medical irresponsibility are used to justify additional management initiatives, such as the Northern Territory Emergency Response. Through discussions of food and nutrition, attitudes regarding race, economy, and governmentality are embodied and deployed. However, these meanings are not unequivocally accepted by Warlpiri people.

Even though the bulk of the population in Lajamanu was born after rationing ended, food distribution, then and now, is a vehicle through which negative attitudes toward government interference in the lives of Aboriginal people are expressed. Not surprisingly, many Lajamanu residents asserted that the Northern Territory Emergency Response reinstated rationing in the twenty-first century. Some believed that limiting Aboriginal access to cash signaled that the government had yet to abandon its policy of assimilation. Catherine confidently stated that the Intervention was an attempt to encourage Aboriginal people to abandon reciprocity. Like many others in Lajamanu, she complained that because of "sharing" in the community, food was often "hard to keep." Adele nevertheless saw reciprocity as an important strategy that allowed people to have access to resources in times of scarcity. Determined that the government would not be successful in its attempts to change the behaviors of Aboriginal people, she said, "They want to make us like *kardiya* but they can't."

White Afflictions, Aboriginal Remedies

Although rationing might not have had the desired effect of instilling white Australian values in the Aboriginal population, the history of food distribution played a significant role in the lives of Warlpiri people. When older residents recalled the early years of the community, lining up in front of the administrative offices to receive rations was commonly discussed. Although any food introduced by non-Aboriginal settlers could be termed *kardiya-kurlangu* or "belonging to white people," this label is particularly applied to items that are associated with rations or their related products: white flour, bread, beef, meat pies, tea, sugar, and cordial (a syrupy beverage). Borne out of the economic, political, and historical realities that structure race relations in Australia, food categories embody ethnic difference. While foods are good to think, they are also explicitly linked to disease through medical dialogues of nutrition.

Across the Northern Territory, the label "white" or *kardiya* is not only applied to foods but also to the diseases that these foods are thought to trigger, particularly chronic lifestyle illnesses (Beck 1985, 84; Nathan and Leichleitner 1983, 134; Reid 1983, 134; Saggers and Gray 1991, 57;

Willis 1985, 28). An older Warlpiri woman commented, "Because of all that *kardiya* food, like beef, *yapa* are getting really sick *kardiya* way." Diabetes is widely recognized as a white disease, its cause being attributed to the consumption of white food such as processed sugar (Devitt and McMasters 1998; Humphery, Dixon, and Marrawal 1998; Saethre 2005; Scrimgeour, Rowse, and Lucas 1997). Warlpiri people claim that if non-Aboriginal people had not distributed their food, either through ration stations decades ago or the store today, then Aboriginal people would not be suffering from such high rates of disease. Prior to contact Warlpiri people did not have access to processed sugars and it is assumed that they would not have suffered from diabetes. As one man explained, "We say that diabetes is from *kardiya* because we didn't get sick like that before they came." Aboriginal people across the Northern Territory share this view. Humphery, Dixon, and Marrawal (1998, 46) remark that, "almost all our Aboriginal informants stated quite firmly that Aboriginal people did not suffer from diabetes before the European invasion of Australia."

In contrast to *kardiya* foods purchased at the shop, Aboriginal or *yapa* foods are hunted and gathered from the bush. Warlpiri people divide foods into three categories: *kuyu*, *miyi*, and *pama*. Men usually hunt *kuyu*, or meat, although women may kill small animals and reptiles as they forage for bush vegetables, *miyi*. *Pama* denotes delicacies such as witchetty grubs as well as honey ants and bush honey, the latter of which are prized for their sweetness. Warlpiri people attribute the strength and vitality of their ancestors to a constant diet of bush foods. William recounted a story of how his grandfather was able to walk long distances across the desert without resting because he ate bush meat. William concluded, "He was strong from living in the desert and having that bush [food]. Now everyone is weak, soft, not like before." The traditional lifestyle led by Aboriginal people before the colonial encounter is often spoken of as a healthy and prosperous time for Warlpiri people compared to their current circumstances.

When evaluating white and Aboriginal foods, Warlpiri people often use nutrition to illustrate difference. Not only is kangaroo meat considered to be healthier than beef, chicken, or pork, only fat from *kardiya* meat is blamed for causing ill health. Larry asserted, "Bullock fat makes you sick but I get strong eating [kangaroo] fat. It is good for us *yapa*." Similar attitudes are also demonstrated in regards to sweet foods. For instance, Warlpiri remark that bush honey made by native bees does not cause diabetes like foods containing refined sugar. One male diabetic said,

"That sweet food from the store makes me sick but *yapa* food makes me [good]. [Bush honey] is sweet but it doesn't make you sick. It makes you [good]." Both bush honey and bush meats are considered to promote general well-being even though the former is sweet, like the sugar which Warlpiri people blame for causing diabetes, and the latter contains fat, like meats which Warlpiri people blame for causing cardiovascular disease.

Aboriginal foods are also praised for their curative properties. While leaves and sap from plants, often referred to as bush medicines, are used to heal physical complaints, any foodstuff harvested from the bush is considered to aid general health. Consequently, all bush foods act as medicines. Subsisting on a diet of these foods is viewed by many as an effective way to treat illnesses, such as diabetes, that result from eating *kardiya* food. As one man sitting outside the shop eating a meat pie remarked, "If you have diabetes, *yapa* [food] will make you right." Echoing these remarks, George commented, "We have to follow our culture, real way, and eat bush [foods]. That is the only way we can beat these *kardiya* diseases." George felt that if his diabetic wife ate more bush foods and fewer sugars her condition would disappear. Like many people in Lajamanu, George supported his position by stating that medical researchers had scientifically proven that eating bush foods ends diabetes. Although he could not name the title of the published work or any of the specific data, George claimed to have spoken to medical researchers as they were gathering data in Lajamanu.[1]

The language of science, saturated fats, and calories frame activities and geography. Through nutritional narratives, procuring food from the countryside is tied to medical benefits. Michael often endorsed setting up remote "health camps" far away from Lajamanu where access to foods high in fat and sugar would be dramatically reduced and bush food consumption would be increased. In contrast to the bush Lajamanu is often described as an environment that is dirty and polluted, full of hardship and chronic illness. A diabetic asserted, "This disease I have is because I sit down in one place too much. Before, when my people were walking around, hunting, we were healthy and strong. Now we are sick because we drive motorcars and eat rubbish." The current conditions of life, economy, and settlement are blamed for high rates of illness. The path to improved health outcomes requires rejecting the community in favor of the bush. Christopher repeatedly stated that it is only through an abandonment of non-Aboriginal food sources and a subsequent embracing of bush foods that health, particularly for diabetics, will improve. Consequently, statements stressing the nutritional value of local foods have influenced the way in which subsistence activities are conceptualized.

As Warlpiri people often assert, research has shown that native meats and vegetables contain higher levels of vitamins and lower levels of fat and sugar than most foods available at the store (Latz 1995; Naughton, O'Dea, and Sinclair 1986). O'Dea (1983; 1985) found that once rates of hunting and gathering were increased, diabetics from Western Australia saw a marked improvement in all of the abnormalities of diabetes and a reduction in a number of risk factors for cardiovascular disease.[2] She (O'Dea 1985, 99) writes, "a mere seven weeks of 'traditional' life-style were sufficient to substantially reverse a disease which took years to develop." Consequently, government and medical professionals also embrace the consumption of bush foods as a method of reducing rates of chronic ill health. Through nutritional information posters and instructional materials for Aboriginal people and health educators, the Northern Territory Department of Health (1995a; 1998a; 2002) encourages eating bush foods as a way of improving health and strength. Shoppers purchasing food at the store are confronted by large signs proclaiming, "Bush Foods Are Best."

Representing a link to the past and the land, bush foods are at the center of the health debate. Hunting and gathering are not only methods of obtaining a meal; these acts are often cast as tangible representations of traditionality. Through subsistence Warlpiri people are connected to their ancestors as well as the land that they occupy. In Australia hunting and gathering have become icons of Aboriginal action that highlight pervasive notions regarding remoteness, Aboriginality, and health. Statements and debates assessing the value of eating bush foods are also statements and debates assessing the value of performing Aboriginality. Furthermore, the health benefits of hunting and gathering have been invoked to argue for government funding of outstations, small settlements set up in the bush well away from communities. Despite being removed from medical facilities of any kind, outstations are thought to be healthier because people practice cultural activities—such eating bush foods—while restricting access to *kardiya* commodities like alcohol (Kowal 2010). While research indicates that outstations can provide ecological, economic, and social benefits (Altman 2003), there does not seem to be any conclusive data confirming that the health of outstation residents is consistently better than that of those living in communities.[3]

Food, nutrition, and chronic illness provide a vehicle through which Indigenous attitudes toward Indigeneity, colonization, and contemporary ethnic relations are expressed. In the Americas, Indigenous groups similarly employ the language of ethnicity to structure food narratives (Graham 2002; Roy 2006; Tom-Orme 1993). Diabetes is associated with the consumption of commercial foods introduced by white colonizers and the subsequent loss of Indigenous traditions (Garro 2000; Garro and Lang 1993; Lang 2006; Tom-Orme 1993). Regularly distributed by the United States government to Native American nations, rations were also exchanged for land in some instances (Jackson 1993). Like Aboriginal people, Native Americans assert that they did not suffer from diabetes prior to their encounters with white settlers and governments. Illness and the foods held responsible for it are explicitly connected to the abandonment of traditional life and the conditions of modernity. As Garro and Lang (1993, 322) write, "Foods and foodways constitute complex codes for social relations and symbols of cultural identity and change, and as they are linked to aspects of health and illness, provide salient imagery in which to demarcate community and cultural boundaries." Transcending nutritional and economic value, foods embody social and economic relations between Indigenous and non-Indigenous people. Medical narratives draw from these meanings to recast ill health in terms of these relationships.

Tying together food, nutrition, chronic illness, history, and geography, Warlpiri people use medical discourse to affirm Aboriginal lifestyles, culture, and traditions prior to contact, while denouncing past and present conditions of settlement. Stressing that medical researchers have proved bush foods are superior to commercial ones, Warlpiri people utilize the language of science and nutrition. Situating biomedicine within a local context, Adams (2002, 217) writes that, "Proof, in this sense, becomes not just a question of epistemology (however important that remains) but rather a question of the way epistemology is made to speak for politics, history, and free markets in a changing world." Although medical discourse has been employed by governments to entrench social ideas and justify political and economic interventions this same tool is wielded differently in the hands of Indigenous people. Warlpiri individuals marshal existing medical narratives—signs in the store proclaiming "Bush Foods Are Best" and government posters urging Aboriginal people to hunt and gather—to transform foods into their own commentary on ethnic relations. While the government invokes nutrition as a basis for health policies, Warlpiri people rework these ideas to demonstrate the pathology of white control and the vitality of Aboriginality.

The Store

Food is not only a symbol of ethnicity; it is also a commodity necessary for survival. On a daily basis Aboriginal people in Lajamanu procure, exchange, and consume a variety of foodstuffs. While still grounded in social relationships, the realities of materiality are negotiated differently from notional representations. As Jackson (1996, 34) writes, "The meaning of practical knowledge lies in what is accomplished through it, not in what conceptual order may be said to underlie or precede it." The narratives of Lajamanu residents toward food and food distribution often ignore the reality that people do enjoy the ease and convenience of food purchased from the store and takeaway. Considerations such as ease of preparation, income cycles, and social obligations are not reflected in most discourse regarding the value of Aboriginality and pre-contact lifestyles. To contextualize the way in which food is integrated into the social and economic world that Aboriginal people inhabit, the everyday processes through which meals are obtained and consumed are examined. First, the most popular sources of food in the community, the local shop and takeaway, are explored. Then, the discussion shifts to hunting and gathering as an alternative strategy for securing food and one that is considered to result in health benefits. I argue that whether food is purchased or hunted, the act of eating is constrained by similar factors, including income, cost, availability, and a desire to avoid excessive reciprocity.

Data suggest that between 80 percent to 95 percent of all food eaten in Aboriginal communities is purchased at the local store and takeaway, which have been acknowledged as playing a crucial role in supplying food to the inhabitants of remote settlements (Brimblecombe and O'Dea 2009, 549; Food and Nutrition Unit 1998, 1; Northern Territory Department of Health 1995b, 5). In Lajamanu, "the shop" was the only source of commercial food in the community. Managed as a unit and housed in a single building complex, food could be purchased from one of three outlets. The main store stocked the largest selection of foods as well as a modest selection of toiletries, clothes, and housewares. Resembling many small shops across Australia, it contained a few aisles of groceries as well as refrigerator and freezer sections. Lying adjacent to the main shop, the takeaway provided prepared meals such as chips, grilled chicken, stew, salads, and sandwiches. The third food outlet, the video shop, sold a limited selection of foods after the main store closed. Although the hours for each store differed, at least one would always be open on weekdays between 10:00 a.m. to 7:00 p.m.

With ration stations gone stores have taken on the role of supplying food to communities and, depending on the perspective, it is possible to see a resemblance between the two (Humphery, Dixon, and Marrawal 1998, 95). Non-Aboriginal management of the store has led some Lajamanu residents to state that Warlpiri people do not have control over the food that the shop sells, just as they had little control over ration allotments.[4] While the store's stock—what was actually on the shelves on any given day—constrained Aboriginal food purchases and consumption, this was not the case for non-Aboriginal workers. Once a week a group of white residents could be seen waiting for the arrival of the refrigerated truck carrying shipments that were ordered directly from the supermarket in Katherine, which offers a much greater selection of foods. The added expense of freight and the requirement of establishing an account with the store in Katherine prohibited the vast majority of Warlpiri people from obtaining food in this manner. Consequently, the store acted as a reminder of racial difference and inequality.

With their purchases often limited to the Lajamanu store, many Aboriginal people criticized the food that it sold and the prices that it charged. There was a consensus that the range of food sold at the shop was too narrow. I was told that store managers purposely stocked a limited selection of food that was of poor quality and lacked nutritional value. Because the shop is the only source of commercial food in the community, residents felt as if they were being held hostage. Many grievances centered on nutrition. A female shopper who was married to a diabetic complained that the shop did not stock a reasonable selection of foods that were low in sugar. Another woman complained, "They got no selection. Everything is the same. Why don't we have nutritious food like [the supermarket in Katherine] here?" There is also a belief that store managers purposely inflate prices to increase their profits.[5] One man summed up many of these sentiments by saying, "That shop charges too much for rubbish food. Those *kardiya* don't understand what *yapa* need."

As many complaints noted, even though basic foods were stocked at the store there was not always a great deal of selection. For instance, often only two varieties of cheese were readily available: tasty and processed. Often only one brand of a product, such as spaghetti noodles and marinara sauce, was also sold. Although the Lajamanu store did not carry the same variety of items a shopper may expect to find in an urban environment, Warlpiri people consumed a relatively narrow range of food. These items such as large buckets of sugar and flour, which consumers in Sydney might have trouble locating at their supermarket, were present in abundance. Given its small size, the shop also stocked a relatively diverse variety of fruits and vegetables which commonly included apples, bananas, nectarines, kiwi fruit, peaches, oranges, snow peas, beans, mushrooms, potatoes, carrots, celery, lettuce, tomatoes, onions, garlic, zucchini, pumpkins, squash, broccoli, and cauliflower. As with other foods, Warlpiri people generally preferred to eat a small selection of the fresh fruits and vegetables available. Apples were particularly popular but were expensive and sold out quickly.

Although Warlpiri people complained that the shop did not stock nutritious foods, this was not the case. For those wishing to make healthy food choices, wholegrain bread, sugar free cordial, and low fat milk were available. Items containing fewer than 10 grams of sugar and 7.5 grams of fat per 100 grams were labeled with a yellow tag as healthier choices. Some of these foods included canned spaghetti, canned pineapple, canned meat, and assorted dehydrated soup mixes. However, I was told that few people chose items based on these signs. In many cases, familiarity superseded nutritional considerations. For instance, when I asked one older man why he did not eat wholegrain bread as a healthier alternative to white bread he replied, "White bread is what we eat. All the way back in the rationing days, it was what we had. It is proper food." Noting the frequency with which flour, tea, sugar, and chops are consumed, Musharbash (2004, 15) writes, "It is what Warlpiri people at Yuendumu are used to and know as staples since ration depot and communal soup kitchen times." Foods that are now considered to contribute to heart disease and diabetes are simply what many people are accustomed to eating. Growing up on a diet of meat, white bread, and sugary tea has led many residents to continue to consume these foods almost exclusively, despite a range of alternatives sold at the local shop and statements stressing a desire to eat healthier foods. Consequently, the era of rations continues to exert a profound influence on the food choices of Warlpiri people today.

The store was also criticized for its food prices, which were significantly higher than those in urban centers, due, in part, to high freight costs. In its yearly survey, the Northern Territory Department of Health (2008b, 8) estimated that on average it cost 27 percent more to purchase the same basket of food in remote stores in the Katherine region than at a Darwin supermarket, but my own calculations indicate that in Lajamanu this figure is higher. White sugar and cordial, both popular items, cost almost twice as much in Lajamanu, while the price disparity of fresh broccoli was even greater. The high cost of food, coupled with the low earning of residents, led to a large percentage of the family income being spent on food. Correlating the average salary of a family of six with food prices, the Northern Territory Department of Health (2008b, 9) estimated that since 1998 approximately 35 percent of household money in remote Aboriginal communities was spent on food from the store, but some researchers disagree, arguing that government figures underestimate this proportion (Scrimgeour, Rowse, and Lucas 1997, 38). Consequently, income patterns often structure food acquisition.

The two-week income cycle largely determines when and how much food can be purchased. In Lajamanu, as in many Aboriginal communities, there is no meal planning or budgeting from week to week. Income is used for immediate consumption and not for saving (Peterson 1991; Stewart 1997, 84). Food expenditure can be as much as five times higher on days when income is received (Rowse et al. 1994, 65). As a result Aboriginal Territorians often live on a cycle of feast and famine (Povenelli 1993, 178; Scrimgeour, Rowse, and Lucas 1997, 52). The feast occurs during either pay week or benefits week, when large amounts of money are spent to buy food. While pay cycles for some family members coincided, others did not, with some receiving paychecks on differing weeks. As most residents rely on government payments, it is these cycles that impact the community the most. After benefits are received, the Lajamanu store is particularly crowded with shoppers. On one payday I found myself in line behind Daisy, a woman who was raising five children. Like many other women shopping for their families, she was pushing two trolleys filled with food including a10-kilogram bucket of flour, five bottles of cordial, several kilograms of meat, five loaves of bread, five tins of stew, several cans of baked beans, a few boxes of tea, a few apples, a head of cauliflower, milk powder, and a tin of sugar. Daisy explained that she was pleased to once again have money to purchase food that was now in short supply at her home. She said simply, "We are hungry."

Money is often depleted after only a few days. Once income has been exhausted, the famine cycle begins. Lajamanu residents refer to this as "my low week."[6] During this period, a family may not possess enough money to buy even basic necessities, having already spent their entire fortnightly pay. The primary method of obtaining much needed food during "my low week" is to seek assistance from family members through demand sharing. One popular strategy was to seek out individuals on an alternate pay cycle. If an individual is hungry and sees a relative with food, it is common practice to request a share. It is generally considered rude or greedy to refuse a request if in possession of the food item being demanded. Hungry individuals often wait outside the store hoping to spot a kinsman leaving with food. Eager relatives are then capable of appropriating and consuming as much as half of the purchase. As I was helping Daisy load her purchase into her brother's car, a classificatory sister who had been sitting on the grass across from the store approached her and said, "I am hungry. Give me food. You have too much." Daisy reached into her bag and withdrew a couple of loaves of bread and a kilogram of meat. Once her "sister" had departed, Daisy said, "All the time they expect us to feed them and they never take no for an answer. It's no good. They need to get a job like us to buy their own food and not come here hungry all the time."

While demand sharing is the norm, people nevertheless complain about what are perceived to be excessive requests or "humbug." A phrase that one hears often in Lajamanu and across the Northern Territory is "too much humbug." As Heil (2006, 103) notes, "This social support and obligation is continuous but it is often also exhausting and demanding, and impossible to be escaped. . . ." The high cost of food coupled with the chronically low income of community residents motivates many Aboriginal people to attempt to circumvent or reduce requests to share purchased food. Although demand sharing is an important tool for maintaining social relationships, many residents are already responsible for feeding those at home and do not have the funds to support non-household members. Encouraging people to avoid demand sharing, chronic poverty places sociality under stress (Heil and Macdonald 2008, 314). Frequent requests or those for large items can lead to anger and resentment (Musharbash 2009, 144). Consequently, food is both a source of association and irritation. Chronicling the complexities of Warlpiri sociality, Musharbash (2009, 145) characterizes demand sharing as "one of many social practices of testing, establishing, maintaining and breaking relationships; however the subtleties of the actual relationships are worked and reworked also in more intricate and more obliquely expressed ways." Exchange is negotiated via a range of implicit and explicit tactical maneuvers.

The desire to avoid giving away large portions of purchased food affects spending choices. I was told that shopping on the day that checks are received was one strategy for reducing demands for food. Because other members of the community are also receiving income, it is assumed that fewer people will be asking for food, allowing shoppers to return home with a larger amount of their purchase intact. In addition to choosing days and times when it is believed fewer people will be demanding food, shopping trips are ideally kept to a minimum. Residents attempt to purchase as much as possible when money is received. In a further attempt to prevent losing a meal and the money it took to purchase it, provisions are consumed rapidly. Expensive or particularly sought after items, such as fresh fruit, are eaten almost immediately for fear that others will appropriate them. These strategies further reinforce the fortnightly pattern of feast and famine.

Demands of reciprocity do not end once food is taken home. Storing and preparing meals each posed challenges. In Lajamanu, the locks on front doors are often broken, leaving houses open to intruders. Residents are concerned that if left unguarded their food would be pilfered. When this occurred, it was considered impolite to confront perpetrators or demand restitution. Nevertheless, these incursions could lead to lingering resentments. After his mother-in-law took over A\$200 in food while he was visiting friends, Martin became extremely frustrated. Angry that he had lost a great deal of food that would be difficult to replace, Martin nevertheless acknowledged that he could not confront her about the theft because of the prohibitions restricting contact between a man and his mother-in-law. To prevent this from occurring again, Martin installed padlocks on his pantry, refrigerator, and freezer, a common practice in the community. However, even with access to his storage facilities restricted, Martin was often exposed to demands of reciprocity when he attempted to prepare a meal. Like many in the community Martin's home lacked a working stove and oven.[7] His family relied on a small hotplate, but without sufficient cooking facilities, preparing food entailed building a fire and cooking outside or using a functioning oven or stove at a relative's home. Both options often require reciprocity. In the first instance, passers-by could demand a share of the visible food being cooked. In the second, relatives may expect to be fed because their cooking apparatus was being used. On those occasions that Martin or his wife required a full stovetop or oven to prepare a meal, a portion was always given to the household that provided the equipment.

In contrast to food sold from the shop, which must often be cooked, items bought from the takeaway could be consumed immediately. Situated next to the main store, the takeaway serves typical Australian fast food like sandwiches, chips, meat pies, chicken wings, hamburgers, small pizzas, dim sims, and candy, in addition to rice and vegetables, kangaroo stew, and salads. As in the case of the shop, Lajamanu residents repeatedly complained about the food sold at the takeaway, its prices, and the way in which it was managed. Takeaway food, in particular, was believed to cause heart disease. While a few healthy options like salad were sold, the majority of food contained large amounts of sugar, processed carbohydrates, or fat. Older men often encouraged younger ones to hunt for kangaroo instead of buying steak pies at the takeaway. Yet despite these statements, the takeaway is an extremely popular source of food both in Lajamanu and other Aboriginal communities across the Northern Territory. Research shows that in some communities 69 percent of all food transactions occurred at the takeaway (Rowse et al. 1994, 64).

Unlike the store where shoppers spend large amounts of money during a single visit, patrons of the takeaway usually purchase only a single meal of pre-cooked food. When compared to food from the shop, takeaways provided a more effective method for circumventing reciprocity. Whereas shoppers exiting the store are often carrying large boxes of clearly visible food, those leaving the takeaway possess only a small bag or two and emerge to the side of the main shop. Given the vehicle traffic, people do not congregate by the exit of the takeaway, as they do at the shop. The bags containing chips, meat pies, or sodas are often placed discreetly under a seat of a car or otherwise out of view. Intended for immediate consumption, there is no need for functional cooking facilities or a long-term storage location. The concealed food can be easily taken to a location for sharing with a limited number of family members or eaten alone. Data confirm that the majority of the food bought from community takeaways is not shared (Scrimgeour, Rowse, and Lucas 1997, 38).

The purchasing and distribution of food is a meaningful act that is constrained by the socio-economic context of the community. Choosing to eat at the takeaway is a strategy. Given the pervasive conditions of life in remote Aboriginal communities—lack of work, reliance on welfare payments, high cost of food, poorly maintained homes, and absence of reliable cooking facilities—the takeaway provides a source of food that reduces exposure to demands. Unfortunately, prepared food generally has higher levels of fat, sugar, and salt. Despite possessing knowledge of dietary guidelines, nutritional concerns take a back seat to social and economic ones. While George, Christopher, and Michael complained about the unhealthy food served at the takeaway, they continued to regularly patronize it nonetheless.

Hunting and Gathering

While numerous constraints are involved in purchasing food, this is not the only source of sustenance in the community. Hunting and gathering are an important alternative to eating at the takeaway. One strategy to improve health encourages Aboriginal people to supplement their diet of commercial foods with those that have been hunted or gathered from the bush. Warlpiri people affirm the nutritional and social value of bush foods but this has not prompted Lajamanu residents to consume them in place of commercial foods. Although bush foods are praised throughout the Northern Territory, they comprise a diminishing portion of daily food intake (Bird, Bird, and Parker 2005; Stewart 1997). As in the case of the shop, economics and reciprocity impact the frequency of hunting and gathering. Most subsistence activities in the bush require larger amounts of resources, particularly cash, than purchasing food from the store. Given the desirability of bush foods, they are generally shared with greater numbers of people. Consequently, the high costs and inconveniences associated with hunting make bush foods an unrealistic alternative to processed ones.

By far the most valued food item in Lajamanu is meat. "Give me *kuyu* [meat]" is a common refrain. While meat was regularly purchased from the store, bush meat was much more highly prized. Consequently, hunting trips were organized as often as possible. In addition, individuals driving between communities would often depart late, spending the afternoon searching for game before camping along the road and continuing their journey the following day. Large animals such as kangaroos, bustards, and emus are pursued exclusively by men using rifles. Of these, kangaroo is the most sought-after meat. George stressed that he hunted for both cultural and medical reasons. While he enjoyed the taste of kangaroo meat, he also extolled the health benefits that such a diet conferred. On average he organized a dedicated hunting trip approximately once every two months. Leaving the community in the morning, an entire day would be spent locating, killing, butchering, and cooking game. While every hunt was unique, I will describe one expedition that is representative of many of my experiences.

George knocked on my door at ten in the morning. A hunting party was about to depart and he knew I would want to come along. After putting on my boots, I climbed into his Toyota Troop Carrier, which already contained five other men ranging in age from seventeen to thirty. I enjoyed hunting with George, in part because he drove a sturdy four-wheel drive vehicle that was well-maintained. Hunting almost always involved driving off-road to search for game. While some people attempted this in sedan cars, it often led to becoming stranded in loose sand or breaking down.[8] Given the cost, very few people could afford four-wheel drive vehicles, including George. His Toyota was a work vehicle. Consequently, it was regularly serviced and possessed a spare tire, unlike many vehicles in the community.

While George's employer allowed him to take the vehicle hunting, George was responsible for purchasing fuel for these trips. After I took my seat in the Toyota, George informed me that our next stop was the petrol station next to the shop. As men will regularly travel well over a hundred kilometers on a typical hunting trip, adequate fuel was essential. After arriving at the petrol pump, George stated that it was his "my low week" and he had no money. Could I purchase the fuel? As petrol prices in Lajamanu are well above the national average, fuelling a vehicle is an expense that few people could regularly afford. Having accompanied George on other hunting trips, this request did not come as a surprise. Before leaving my house, I had slipped A$100 into my pocket to cover expenses such as this. While I fuelled the Toyota, the other men went into the takeaway to buy food. George remained in the driver's seat, requesting two steak pies, chips, and a bottle of soda.

With our purchases complete, George stated a few preparations still needed to be made before we could leave Lajamanu. A fortnight earlier, George had loaned his own rifle to a kinsman only to have it returned broken. George lamented that he was unable to fix it himself and would have to take it to town on his next visit. Consequently, we needed to borrow a rifle. We began driving around the community in an attempt to locate men who owned firearms. This was not an easy task. Rifles were expensive and many men could not afford them. To legally own a firearm, furthermore, it was necessary to possess a shooter's license. This required the applicant to pass a test in English, submit to an eye exam, and show proof of a secure storage space meeting government specifications. Consequently, firearms were in short supply in Lajamanu.

Our first stop was at home of a kinsman, Mark. It was empty. Hoping to find him visiting his sister, we drove to her home. She informed us that he had left for Yuendumu a day earlier. One of the men present suggested that we ask Ian. Arriving at his home we found that it too was empty. We eventually located him at the store. He informed us that his rifle had already been loaned to someone else, but recommended a third choice, Bruce. Once again we began searching the community. Finally, we located Bruce, who agreed to loan George his rifle in return for a portion of the hunt. Finding a rifle had taken over two hours. But we were still not ready to depart the community. George needed bullets. However, it was Saturday and the shop had already closed for the day. It would not re-open until Monday. The bullets would have to be borrowed as well. Once again we drove around the community. It took considerably less time to procure bullets, but George had to promise to distribute more meat in repayment. More than three hours after George knocked on my door, we left Lajamanu.

Heading south, we began following the main road, which was unpaved and corrugated. As we drove George discussed the health benefits of eating bush foods and encouraged the young men present to avoid patronizing the takeaway. Conversations such as this were a common occurrence on hunting trips. After driving for about an hour, George veered off into the bush. It took another half an hour of weaving around acacia trees and termite mounds before a group of three kangaroos was spotted. Driving slowly, George eased the Toyota toward the animals. Once within range, the engine was turned off and the rifle was loaded. George took aim and fired. The shot missed its mark. The target quickly bounded away but two other kangaroos remained. George reloaded and fired again. This time a kangaroo jerked and fell to the ground, while the third animal fled into the bush. We drove to the injured kangaroo. It was a small female. She was wounded but the bullet would not kill her immediately. George instructed one of the young men to hand me a wooden club resembling a small baseball bat. It was my task to break the animal's neck.

After the kangaroo was killed, we tied the carcass to the top of the roof rack and set off once more. Over the next two hours another kangaroo and a bustard were shot. During our journey, a curious dingo, no doubt attracted by the blood dripping down the side of the Toyota, trotted behind us briefly before moving off in search of its own prey. It was a very successful trip.

Before returning to the community, we needed to cook the game. While ovens and stoves are used to prepare *kardiya* meat, bush meat is always cooked in the ground. George knew of a place beside the main road where the soil was loose and easy to dig, perfect for fashioning an earth oven. We were still a few kilometers away when a loud bang was heard. The left rear tire had been punctured. I was silently grateful that George always carried a spare. However, it soon became apparent that there was another problem. George had loaned his jack to a kinsman. There was no way to raise the vehicle. After considering the problem, a solution was found. Kicking over several termite mounds, we piled the rubble in a heap in front of the flat tire. George carefully drove the car forward until the wheel was directly on top of the mound. More rubble was now placed under the carriage of the Toyota to support the vehicle in its raised position. Using the club and a tire iron, the first mound was removed from under the flat and we were able to change the tire. With the spare in place, George drove forward and the rubble supporting the vehicle collapsed. We were on our way once again.

Once we arrived at the main road, preparing the oven was relatively straightforward but time-consuming. One group of men dug a hole approximately a meter deep while another collected firewood. George removed the entrails of the animals while I plucked the bustard. Examining the kangaroo carcasses, George commented that the animals possessed an exceptional amount of fat. The fat, he added, would not only make the meat taste better, it would make him strong. Referring to the high fat content, George said, "If this was *kardiya kuyu*, I might die. But this is *yapa kuyu* so I will be right." A fire was lit and allowed to burn until only coals remained. The carcasses were placed on top of the coals in the pit and covered with earth. While we waited for the meat to cook, the sun set and the stars rose. When we finally drove in to Lajamanu, it was after ten in the evening. Despite the late hour many people were anxiously awaiting our return. The families of those on the trip as well as those who had contributed the rifle and bullets wanted a share of the meat. In addition, others in the community had heard about the expedition and were hoping to obtain a portion as well. Within fifteen minutes all of the meat was claimed and distributed. George joked that there wasn't enough left for him. While George had spent over twelve hours hunting, it only provided one meal.

Although hunting is an important activity and one that is considered to engender better health, George, like most men in Lajamanu, talks about its value more than he actually does it. The practical difficulties of hunting often limited the number of trips that he made. This hunting trip was not unique. While the delays and complications varied, they always occurred. On one occasion, when hunting with another family, a spare tire had to be borrowed before leaving the community. On another, the petrol station was closed and the trip had to be postponed altogether. Even if the arrangements go smoothly, the amount of time it takes to hunt, kill, and cook a kangaroo, or any large game, is several hours and can easily take much longer. In addition to the lengthy procedure, the borrowed materials will incur social obligations that are repaid with a share of the meat. Game is generally not stored after it is cooked and any leftovers are quickly taken by others. As a result, a hunting trip will only yield a single meal. Bush meats may be healthier, but hunting is a long and complex procedure that requires having access to resources difficult to find in Lajamanu: a reliable car, a gun, a hunting license, money to purchase petrol and bullets, and a reasonable amount of free time.[9] These constraints have been noted to limit hunting activities across the Northern Territory (Bird, Bird, and Parker 2005; Povenelli 1993; Stewart 1997). In comparison to hunting, buying chips and meat pies from the takeaway only takes a few minutes and is much cheaper.

Like hunting, gathering is also a time-consuming enterprise. While men travel long distances in search of meat, families must also travel in search of vegetable foods (*miyi*) and delicacies (*pama*). A car is almost always needed to search for bush vegetables. Although many edible plants can be found in the immediate vicinity of Lajamanu, most residents will not consume them. *Ngayaki* or *wanakiji* (*Solanum chippendalei*), commonly called bush tomato, grows on a thorny shrub about a meter high on the roadside leading into Lajamanu. These plants are not used for food because they grow too close to the community and are considered unhealthy. As one woman related, "There is too much rubbish around Lajamanu. It makes that *miyi* rubbish one—no good to eat. It is much better to go a little bit long way." Sites just outside this perimeter, which are ideal for foraging, are often over-picked. As a result, gathering activities are generally not conducted within a nine-kilometer radius of the community, making a vehicle essential. Since men control many of the vehicles in the community, women may have a more difficult time locating transportation.

One non-meat food that is often discussed as being particularly beneficial to health is bush honey or *ngarlu*. Bush honey is produced by small wild bees, which deposit nectar in hollow branches of trees. The bees do not possess stings, making the collection of bush honey a painless event. Like most bush food, *ngarlu* is believed to aid general well-being and is considered to be an effective treatment for diabetes. I spoke to two diabetics who ceased taking medication to control the disease, vowing instead to eat *ngarlu* regularly. However, for many people in the community, consuming *ngarlu* is rare. As with hunting for kangaroo, collecting *ngarlu* was a lengthy venture.

I left Lajamanu on a Saturday with George, his wife, Margaret, and several others, including their children. The weekend was usually the only time that both George and Margaret had time off work to engage in hunting and gathering activities. After driving approximately sixty kilometers north of Lajamanu, we stopped in an area known for its plentiful supply of *ngarlu*. We then walked through the bush for about an hour until Margaret's younger sister located a tree with a number of bees flying around one of its branches. However, the bough was a considerable distance off the ground and we did not possess a ladder. We abandoned the tree and started looking again. More than two hours passed before we identified a tree that was the suitable height. George drove the Toyota under the branch and pointed out the entrance to the honey cache, called the *milpa* or eye. There is no wax comb, only a thick mass of honey topped by a small pollen residue called a *jurru* or head. The most effective method of harvesting honey is to first sever the entire branch from the tree. George had brought a saw and two axes for this purpose. The men climbed onto the roof rack of the Toyota and chopped away at the branch, carefully ensuring that the honey cache was not damaged. It took more than an hour to remove the bough. Placing it on the ground, the branch was split open and the *ngarlu* was eagerly scooped out and eaten. Each person received about five tablespoons of honey. Despite the effort, the *ngarlu* provided a negligible amount of the food intake for the day. Earlier, while waiting to locate a honey tree, the group had consumed a large lunch of white bread, sugary tea, and grilled meat.

Whether food is hunted, gathered, purchased, or distributed, these acts are constrained by the social and economic context of the community. While the fortnightly cycle constrains personal income, these monies are nevertheless used to establish and maintain sociality. One way in which this is accomplished is through hunting and gathering activities as well as sharing food. While the Australian state is in control of distributing monies, Aboriginal agency does play a role in determining the use and redistribution of these resources. Food is simultaneously a reminder of the economic realities that structure the lives of Indigenous people and a statement of Indigenous identity.

On the drive back to Lajamanu, George and the others discussed the value of eating bush honey. Many of those present simultaneously affirmed the cultural and nutritional value of bush foods while complaining that takeaway and other white foods were toxic. Food was not only a source of health; it was also an entity through which the social world was embodied. Redeploying the language of nutrition, the shop and sugar acted as metaphors of race. Through narratives of white foods causing white diseases, which are then effectively cured by eating Aboriginal foods, Warlpiri people are able to contest the history, economy, and social relations of remote communities. Medical narratives of health and illness re-imagine earlier discourses that stressed the pathology of Aboriginality. Instead of an avenue to employment and civilization, colonial and commercial food distribution has come to connote the negative impact of government interference, while the efficacy bush foods affirms the value of Aboriginal identity.

Significantly, these narratives of resistance are made possible though illness. Food and nutrition have become noteworthy topics as a result of the persistently high rates of obesity, diabetes, malnutrition, and chronic disease. These conditions severely impact life expectancies and, in so doing, create a platform from which powerful statements about Indigeneity can be made. Linking narratives of improved nutrition to hunting and gathering, Aboriginal practices are acknowledged as beneficial by both Aboriginal and non-Aboriginal people. In contrast to views that portray demand sharing (and other Aboriginal practices) as an impediment to personal and family economic advancement (Kowal and Paradies 2010; Peterson and Taylor 2003; Sutton 2009), the endorsement of hunting and gathering constitutes a powerful counter-narrative. Widely reported in the media and generally supported by medical staff and government officials, assertions regarding the benefits of eating bush foods visibly cast adherence to Aboriginality as restorative. Furthermore, the importance of continued hunting and gathering to Aboriginal health can be used to argue for important resources such as control over access and management of local environments. Being sick is not only a physical condition or a system of meaning, it is also a practical tool that can be tactically wielded to gain recognition and rights from a nation that routinely marginalizes Aboriginal people.

CHAPTER 3
Contemporary Cosmologies

In the brief respite between the disruption of Christmas, when the shop and only source of food in the community could be closed for as many as five days, and the upcoming initiation ceremonies, many people tried to relax.[1] George had arrived at my home, accompanied by his self-proclaimed tribe of family members, to unwind and escape the heat by sitting under the air-conditioning and watching a kung fu movie starring Jet Li. Just getting the film had posed a considerable challenge. In an effort to reduce accidental property damage, most individuals are extremely reluctant to loan out any of their own videos. On this occasion, Alex, the owner of the video was out of town. He had driven to Top Springs, three hundred kilometers away, to purchase alcohol. George informed me that Alex had left Lajamanu before sunset in an effort to avoid sighting a UFO. Coinciding with the regular downpours of the rainy season, UFO activity around the community was thought to increase, particularly during the night. George was confident that the distance, alcohol, and fear of UFOs, would keep Alex out all evening. Consequently, he could not object to our borrowing his video.

As I put the videotape in the player and turned off the lights, George asserted that he preferred to watch Asian actors in martial arts films because, "It is *jukurrpa* [Dreaming] for them." We settled back to enjoy the movie but all that appeared on the television screen was a garbled picture. After fast forwarding, we discovered that the Cantonese dialogue could be heard clearly but the picture remained scrambled and the subtitles were not visible at all. I was assured that the cassette was in good condition; consequently, the video player was blamed. George predicted that the heads were dirty. Since my cleaner had disappeared weeks ago, a casualty of a loan, George's son, Donald, left to borrow a substitute from relatives.

While we waited, I prepared tea for everyone. The children, though, were restless and began running around the room. After a few cups were narrowly missed, Carl casually left his seat and slowly moved toward an open window. Looking out into the darkness, he pointed and exclaimed "*kuku* [ghost]." The children lurched to a halt in fear. A few of the adults gave a cursory glance out the window while saying, "*kuku* there" in concerned tones. After the initial shock, the children quickly returned to a normal state and the reckless behavior stopped. To illustrate the danger posed by ghosts, Margaret commented that one of the children present had been ensorcelled by a *kuku* only a few days earlier while swimming late at the creek. The girl had become quite ill, suffering from a high fever and vomiting. Only after a *ngangkari* removed a magic bone did she begin to feel better.

After we had waited for over half an hour, Donald returned offering little in the way of explanation except that his mission was unsuccessful. Silently, we pondered other options. George suggested disassembling the video player and cleaning the heads manually with cotton buds and rubbing alcohol. But once again, I did not possess the necessary supplies. George told me not to worry; I could go to the clinic and ask the nurses for the materials that we needed. Glancing at my watch, I noticed that it was close to midnight. Although the nurses were required to deliver care at all hours if an emergency occurred, I was sure that this did not qualify. I informed George that I was not willing to wake the nurses at this hour. George replied that he had another solution.

George approached the video player in mock seriousness and closed his eyes. A look of calculated concentration came across his face. Cupping his hands over his abdomen, he made a fist. George's eyes opened and concentrating intently, he brought his closed hands to his mouth where he blew on them. Then George moved his fists toward the video player. Small giggles were made from those present. George slowly opened his hands as if he was pushing something into the machine. At first gripping it intensely, he gradually rotated his hands around the video player. As he performed the action he was hardly able to suppress a chuckle himself. Meanwhile, almost everyone present was laughing uncontrollably. Finally, having circumnavigated the machine with his hands, George turned around and shrugged his shoulders in mock resignation. His mouth, however, was stretched into a large grin. George had jokingly used the same technique any *ngangkari* would to diagnose an ill individual.

Aboriginal beliefs regarding sorcery have captivated explorers, researchers, and anthropologists. Writing over a hundred years ago, Spencer and Gillen (1904, 455) typified Aboriginality by noting the ubiquity of magic across the country. Although the lifestyle of Aboriginal peoples has changed dramatically over the last century, "the anthropological literature is skewed toward documenting the presence of 'traditional' beliefs" (Scrimgeour, Rowse, and Lucas 1997, 27). Saggers and Gray (1991, 42) employ Clements' (1932) typology of "primitive medicine" to categorize and explain "traditional" Aboriginal health practices in contemporary Australia. When examining health beliefs, Indigenous cosmologies are often cast as discrete and contrasted with "modern" medical explanations.

In treating tradition as a circumscribed entity, researchers have tended to focus on the ways in which Indigenous cosmologies are deployed to configure and reflect Indigenous social relations. Consequently, conceptions of ghosts, ancestral beings, sorcery, and spiritual illness have been regarded by anthropologists in Australia as a major mechanism through which norms were enforced, uncertainty was explained, and social tensions were diffused (Berndt 1974; Cawte 1965; Elkin 1994; Reid 1983; Roheim 1974; Tonkinson 1978). Cawte's (1974) monograph, *Medicine Is the Law*, succinctly encapsulates this view. Illness provided an idiom through which day-to-day community interactions between individuals, families, and clans could be raised and resolved. While I broadly agree that narratives such as sorcery accusations give voice to collective and individual anxieties, I believe that these anxieties include existing conditions of life in Indigenous communities such as marginalization, governance, and racial difference.

Indigenous cosmologies are not simply relics of the past that exist in isolation. Austin-Broos (1996b, 3) refers to the "inevitable recasting of cosmology in the face of a changing world." Examining spirituality among Arrernte people, she (1996a, 17) notes that there has been an "inter-penetration of ontologies," where devout Aboriginal Christians hold sorcery beliefs without any apparent contradiction. Although Christianity represents a universalizing tendency to a specific doctrine, Aboriginal people are able to appropriate Biblical narratives to address colonization and contemporary social relations (McDonald 2010, 2001). Christianity in Aboriginal communities has been analyzed as the result of a combination of factors including the economy, the state, and Indigenous ideas of personhood (Schwarz 2010a, 66). Rather than examining Christianity in Lajamanu, I wish to apply these lessons to medical narratives. Schwarz (2010b, 72) explores the way in which Aboriginal people recast biomedical diagnoses and procedures in terms of Christianity or sorcery to reclaim "sickness within the Aboriginal domain, creating a semblance of control." I believe that this domain encompasses contemporary experiences of affliction and resistance. An examination of four aspects of Warlpiri spiritual health—the soul, the ability to heal, sorcery, and protective spirits—illustrates that "traditional" notions are firmly entrenched within the "modern" contexts of ethnic identity, genetics, domestic violence, alcohol abuse, chronic illness, and government intervention. Tales of spiritual illness, ghosts, and sorcery continue to permeate Lajamanu, but they are told in an environment of UFO sightings, kung fu movies, and joking attempts to heal a video player using magic.

Souls

Warlpiri cosmology is grounded in the concept of *jukurrpa*. Translated as "Dreaming," "Dream Time," and "Ancestral Time," *jukurrpa* denotes more than these simple glosses indicate. Although encompassing a variety of meanings, *jukurrpa* most commonly denotes a time during which ancestral beings emerged from the earth and roamed the landscape. Dussart (2000, 18) refers to this era as the "Ancestral Present," noting that it is "situated simultaneously in the distant past (*nyuruwiyi*) and in the present (*jalangu*)." *Jukurrpa* can also signify the ancestral beings themselves, who travelled across the countryside, performed tasks, and conducted rituals. As ancestral beings moved throughout the environment and created geographic features, their essences permeated the land. Characterized as "life forces" by Peterson (1969, 27), these essences embody the power of *jukurrpa* and, through the act of conception, form the basis of the soul.

Establishing a link between the individual, land, and sociality, Aboriginal conception beliefs have been extensively studied by anthropologists (Berndt and Berndt 1974; Kaberry 1939; Merlan 1986; Montagu 1974; Munn 1973; Peile 1997; Tonkinson 1978; Wild 1975). For Warlpiri people, the active agents of conception are referred to as *kurruwalpa*, often glossed as "spirit children" in anthropological literature. Manifestations of ancestral power associated with specific sites, *kurruwalpa* are described as mischievous sprites residing in trees, water holes, and caves. Pregnancy is triggered when a *kurruwalpa* shoots the power and essence of *jukurrpa* into the womb of the mother, animating the fetus. At this point, the woman will discover her pregnancy, either through a dream or the onset of physical symptoms. The *jukurrpa* associated with the site at which this event occurs is considered to be the child's natal or conception *jukurrpa*. Although the *jukurrpa* affiliation gained through conception is not given a major expression in ritual, it is important for understanding the spiritual composition of the self and the way in which Warlpiri people are united with the land on which they live. In Warlpiri, the phrase *jukurrpa-warnu*, "belonging to the Dreaming," denotes a birthmark.

Through the act of conception, individuals possess *kuruwarri*. Like the term *jukurrpa*, *kuruwarri* can be employed in a number of different contexts. Munn (1973, 119) states, "The term *guruwari* can be used in a general sense to refer to any visible mark left by an ancestor in the country, and in addition, *guruwari* in the abstract aspect of 'ancestral powers' are lodged in country." *Kuruwarri* is an essence present in the physical environment as well as all tangible instantiations of *jukurrpa*, including rituals, designs, sacred objects, and customary law. In Lajamanu people also referred to *kuruwarri* as embodied in human beings. Through the process of conception and participation in ritual, *kuruwarri* is personified in individuals, linking them to land, ancestors, and expressions of this power.

While *kuruwarri* is unbounded, the *pirlirrpa*—the soul, self, and life force—is individual. The *pirlirrpa* is created as a result of the presence of *kuruwarri* and *kurruwalpa* but is distinct from them. Anchored in the kidneys, the *pirlirrpa* is considered to be the locus of individual physical, spiritual, and emotional experiences. In the Warlpiri language, attitude, volition, and character are often expressed by reference to the *pirlirrpa*. A "cool *pirlirrpa*," *pirlirrpa-walyka*, denotes a feeling of calm or pleasure, while a "strong *pirlirrpa*," *pirlirrpa-pirrjirdi*, indicates confidence or bravery, as does a "comfortable *pirlirrpa*," *pirlirrpa-purlku*. Someone of "two souls," *pirlirrpa-jarra*, is undecided. An unbalanced, disturbed or mentally deficient person is said to be "without a *pirlirrpa*," *pirlirrpa-wangu*.

While the *pirlirrpa* resides in an individual's body, it is not permanently tied to the corporeal self. During sleep, the *pirlirrpa* can leave the body and travel throughout the physical and spiritual environment—attending ceremony, attaining knowledge, or visiting the heavens. Upon waking, the *pirlirrpa* should return to its proper location in the body. However, if a nightmare or other disturbance suddenly rouses the sleeper, the *pirlirrpa* could "slip," usually retreating to the extremities. Consequently, parents rub the faces of their children lightly to wake them, allowing their *pirlirrpa* to enter the body slowly and settle in its proper place. Other startling events, such as an unexpected dog's bark, could similarly cause the *pirlirrpa* to shift inside the body. Consequently, in Warlpiri, a shocked, upset, or frightened individual is referred to as *pirlirrpa jurnta-yani*, literally "*pirlirrpa* away take." Likewise, amazement may also be indicated by the phrase "*pirlirrpa* without location," *pirlirrpa-wangurlu*.

The proper placement and functioning of the *pirlirrpa* is necessary for good health. When the *pirlirrpa* shifts away from its location in the kidneys, the body becomes imbalanced and illness ensues. Symptoms can include fever, aches, nausea, and insomnia. Children are considered to be the most prone to suffering from this type of spiritual illness. If a slipped *pirlirrpa* is left untreated, the symptoms will eventually disappear as the *pirlirrpa* naturally realigns itself. However, most residents reported preferring to shorten their illness experience by having a *ngangkari* shift their *pirlirrpa* back into place.

While ill health can occur because of a slippage of the *pirlirrpa*, a more severe type of spiritual illness results when objects, which I refer to as pathogens, are magically implanted into a victim's *pirlirrpa* through sorcery. The most common pathogens are pointed pieces of bone, called *yarda*, although any sharp object such as wood, pins, and knives could be used. In addition, other objects including snakes, hair string, and stones have also been reported. To embed a pathogen, a ritual is performed by either non-corporeal agents or human sorcerers, which causes the desired object to magically fly through the air until it hits, penetrates, and lodges in the *pirlirrpa* of the victim. Because these rituals involve chanting, most acts of sorcery are colloquially referred to as "being sung." Once afflicted by a pathogen, symptoms often include high fevers, vomiting, confusion, and severe internal pain. Symptoms will progressively worsen and, unless successfully treated by a *ngangkari*, death will ensue.

In Lajamanu, everyday narratives of sorcery and *kuruwarri* are not confined to descriptions of pathogens and natal *jukurrpa*. They also speak to existing social conditions in Australia. Cosmology and etiological beliefs play a central role in situating the individual within a multiethnic environment where racial dichotomies structure the social world. In some contexts, so-called traditional explanations are utilized to vocalize and reconfigure ideas of contemporary ethnic identity, particularly when the boundaries between Aboriginal and non-Aboriginal appear to be transgressed. For instance, seniors often rebuked young men for failing to attend important ceremonies or participate in hunting trips. When this occurred, race and cosmology could be linked. Chiding his grandson, one man said, "You are not really Warlpiri. You have no *kuruwarri*. You are just like *kardiya*." In this statement, *kuruwarri* is not just an embodiment of *jukurrpa*, it is also a metaphor for Aboriginality.

Similarly, notions of sorcery are used to negotiate the social border between Aboriginal and non-Aboriginal. Although there was no clear cosmological doctrine as to why this was the case, I was advised that *kardiya* were immune to spiritual illness. When I first arrived in Lajamanu, I was told that I should consider myself lucky that I did not have to worry about becoming the victim of a sorcerer. Over time, however, this proved not to be the case. After living in the community for 18 months I began suffering from a high fever, vomiting, and stomach cramps. As was often my practice I consulted a *ngangkari*. On previous visits I had been told that I was suffering from a physical disease and advised to go to the clinic. However, on this occasion, a *yarda* was removed from my body. The *ngangkari* stated that I had been ensorcelled by a *kuku* while taking a walk in the early evening. As the story of my illness spread around the community, many people reacted with surprise, given my status as *kardiya*. As time passed I discovered that bewilderment seemed to have been transformed into pride. When Warlpiri people introduced me to others, they remarked that I was the *kardiya* that had been ensorcelled. My illness became a mark of my association with Warlpiri people and acceptance into the social life of the community.

In her examination of the way in which local illness categories and cosmologies are able to facilitate social change, Crandon-Malamud (1997) explores the relationship between disease and identity in the Andes. She contends that through narratives that affirm or deny local etiologies, Andeans socially situate themselves and others. Similarly, racial categories feature in Warlpiri discussions of sorcery, and beliefs about the power of *ngangkari* highlight statements regarding the ubiquity of white illness in Aboriginal communities. These explanations also reflect shifting commitments and ethnic identities.

The Power to Heal

Spiritual illnesses, those affecting the *pirlirrpa*, are exclusively diagnosed and treated by *ngangkari*.[2] While it is theoretically possible for anyone in the community, male or female, young or old, to be a *ngangkari*, in reality, these individuals were invariably male, ranging in age from one year old to over sixty. Despite their healing abilities *ngangkari* do not enjoy a privileged place in community hierarchy nor do they possess unique, sacred, secret knowledge or ritual responsibility.[3] In Lajamanu, *ngangkari* not only lack biomedical training, they do not treat physical illnesses such as cuts, diabetes, or infectious disease, nor do they usually distribute bush medicines, vitamin supplements, or pharmaceuticals.

Exclusively concerned with maintaining the health of the *pirlir-rpa*, *ngangkari* possess *nguwa*, a magical substance that bestows heightened senses as well as the ability to diagnose and heal spiritual disease. Often depicted as a small luminous ball or shining crystal by residents of Lajamanu, Cawte and Kidson (1964, 979) remark that their Warlpiri informants characterized *nguwa* as soft and white. George described his *nguwa* as glowing like a light, adding that it allowed him to see distant objects as well as the radiant *nguwa* of other *ngangkari*. Residing in the abdomen, *nguwa* also makes soft noises, described as resembling those of a ticking clock. George's wife would often complain that his *nguwa* would keep her awake at night with its incessant clicking. While many men in Lajamanu possessed *nguwa*, only those with several balls or pieces were considered to be *ngangkari*.[4] George, his three sons, Carl, Donald, and Mathew, as well as his infant grandson, Alan, had all obtained *nguwa* at some point during their lives.

Nguwa has its origins in the animal world but there is no clear doctrine on its genesis.[5] Most *ngangkari* can identify the animal from which his power was derived. Carl stated that his five pieces of *nguwa* consisted of two from dogs (*maliki*), two from birds (*jurlpu*), and one from an eagle (*warlawurru*). *Ngangkari* are not thought to personify these animals and special dietary restrictions or customary prohibitions do not exist. Although Tonkinson (1978, 107) and Taylor (1977, 33) describe other Aboriginal groups as employing "spirit familiars" to aid in diagnosis and treatment, Warlpiri do not use representations of animals for healing purposes. Nevertheless, *nguwa* does establish a connection between human and animal. For instance, when Carl spotted an eagle flying overhead, he stated that this was a representation of the substance inside him. Although his *nguwa* could be instantiated by a physically present bird, the eagle did not otherwise participate in Carl's life or activities. Animals are only a source of *nguwa* and otherwise play little role in the daily lives of *ngangkari*.

Bestowing a greater awareness of both the physical and spiritual world, *nguwa* heightens the senses of individuals, allowing them to perceive things others cannot, primarily of a spiritual nature, as well as enabling examination of the internal body. One *ngangkari* explained that his *nguwa* made it possible for him to see inside others in a manner similar to that of an x-ray. But unlike x-rays, *nguwa* detects the state of the *pirlirrpa*. Not only does *nguwa* provide the means for healing but also the knowledge required to perform such actions. *Nguwa* directs the *ngangkari* through internal cues. Techniques and procedures are developed in this way, not through a mentoring process. George, describing his own abilities reported, "I just listen to my *nguwa* and it tells me what to do. It's not like university, where you have to study. *Ngangkari* just know." Unlike the powers of sorcerers, those of *ngangkari* cannot be learnt.[6]

For a *ngangkari* to diagnose and treat a disease he must withdraw the *nguwa* from his own body and insert it into that of his patient. Clasping his hands together over his solar plexus, the *ngangkari* extracts a few pieces of *nguwa*, grasping it firmly in his fist. The *ngangkari* often blows into his hands to intensify the *nguwa*'s power. Touching the patient's body, usually the abdomen or back, the *ngangkari* slowly opens his hand to release the *nguwa*. Running his hands over the patient's stomach, chest, neck, and back, the *ngangkari* occasionally stops to firmly press a particular area. During this process, the *nguwa* circulates inside the patient informing the *ngangkari* of the state and location of the patient's *pirlirrpa*. Pathogens, such as *yarda*, feel hot, whereas the healthy body is cool.

If a pathogen is identified, the *ngangkari* directs the *nguwa* to adhere to the object. Then, the healer usually makes a cutting motion with his hand over the location of the bone. Directing his *nguwa* to pull out the object though the invisible incision, the *ngangkari* grasps both in his fist. After returning the *nguwa* to his own body, the *ngangkari* shows the patient what he removed, which is most often a *yarda*. However, younger *ngangkari* no longer display physical pathogens after completing treatment, claiming that these objects are present but invisible. In these instances, the *ngangkari* makes a crushing motion with his hand and then discards the invisible object.

During treatment, the *ngangkari* must ensure that he inserts only a portion of his *nguwa* into the patient, retaining a few pieces for himself. Without a small share of the substance still present in his own body, the *ngangkari* cannot communicate with the *nguwa* inside the patient. Not only will the healer be unable to diagnose or treat the illness, he will lose his powers completely, having transferred them to the patient. Consequently, only those men who have a sufficient amount of *nguwa* to insert a few pieces into a patient while retaining others are called *ngangkari*. While Carl possessed five pieces and was considered to be a *ngangkari*, George was not, having only two. Although the *nguwa* enhanced his senses, allowing George to see spirit beings, he was not strong enough to extract pathogens, which often requires four or more pieces, depending on the strength of the sorcerer.

In addition to its healing ability, *nguwa* also alerts and protects its owner from malevolent forces, such as spirit beings. The ticking of *nguwa* will increase in both frequency and intensity should danger approach, prompting the *ngangkari* to action. Older, more experienced *ngangkari* often use their *nguwa* to drive away *kuku*, by throwing it at them. Although still a boy, Mathew discovered another use for the painful properties of his *nguwa* when Wendy, a young girl, began physically tormenting him. Although she was rarely spooked by the threat of *kuku*, Mathew learned that taking out his *nguwa* and throwing it at Wendy caused her to experience a brief, but sharp, pain. He only had to lay his hand on his stomach and she would quiet down in fear.

Although *ngangkari* did not enjoy special social privileges in Lajamanu, the increased cognitive and defensive abilities that accompanied the possession of *nguwa* motivated many men to attempt to acquire the substance. The primary methods of attaining *nguwa* in Lajamanu are either through contact with a wild animal or a person possessing the substance. Many men reported obtaining *nguwa* while visiting their "country" but the transfer from animal to human can occur almost anywhere in the rural environment. For instance, George first received his *nguwa* when driving back from Katherine. While urinating on the side of the road, he felt an object fall on his head. At first, George believed he had been hit by bird droppings but when he wiped his head, nothing was there. A few days later, he became ill. It was at that moment that he realized a bird had given him *nguwa*. Another Lajamanu resident described receiving *nguwa* while droving cattle across the Northern Territory. He remarked that although he did not see the animal that gave him the substance, he could feel it inside of him. Similarly, a third individual stated that he obtained all but one of his *nguwa* by chance encounters with animals in the bush. One of these occasions occurred while hunting for kangaroos. He had sighted the animal and raised his gun. But before the bullet could be discharged, he felt an object, later identified as *nguwa*, hit his body. The kangaroo quickly bounded away unharmed.

George regularly expressed a wish to have more *nguwa* to make him strong enough to become a *ngangkari* and better resist *kuku*. He commented that Carl was fortunate to possess as many as five pieces. Instead of relying on unpredictable encounters in the bush, it was possible to obtain *nguwa* from another individual. The donor simply inserts the *nguwa* into the recipient's body, but unlike the process of diagnosis, it is not recalled. In many instances where transfers occurred, it was between close family members. For instance, Cawte and Kidson (1964, 981) recount a story of a dying man passing on his healing abilities to his son before his death. In Lajamanu, Jacob, a senior *ngangkari*, described how he first obtained his *nguwa* decades earlier from his mother's brother. Furthermore, exchanging *nguwa* within a family was done without much concern. Sitting around the television at night, I would often hear George's sons ask for *nguwa* to increase their strength. Not long after Alan was born, George placed a piece of his *nguwa* inside the baby. Similarly, George had also given *nguwa* to Donald a few years earlier. *Nguwa*, like food, was the subject of the demands of reciprocity. Social relations were negotiated, in part, through the exchange of healing abilities.

While *nguwa* was often shared within families, not all transfers were consensual. Thefts occurred most often when a *ngangkari* was sick, drunk, or weakened. During diagnosis and treatment, a portion of the patient's *nguwa* could be removed along with that of the healer. Distracted by illness, the victim rarely noticed what had happened until after it was too late. George, for instance, described having his *nguwa* stolen while consulting a healer in a neighboring community. When his *nguwa* returned for no apparent reason, George took steps to ensure it would not be taken again. He gave his sons and grandson small amounts of his *nguwa* making the levels in his body less detectable to thieves. On the occasions when George became very ill, he often discussed transferring his *nguwa* to his sons for safety.

Whether obtained in the bush or from another individual, once *nguwa* has been transferred into the recipient's body, it begins to grow and move throughout the body. If the individual already possessed *nguwa*, this is a relatively easy process. As the *nguwa* becomes mature, the older pieces anchor the newer ones firmly in the solar plexus. However, if the *nguwa* is entering a pristine body, severe headaches and other symptoms will often result. Once its development is complete, it is common to ask another *ngangkari* to shift the *nguwa* into position, which is referred to as being "opened up." At this point, most of the discomfort ceases, although men that have been *ngangkari* for years occasionally experience symptoms. Fixing the position of *nguwa* is also necessary to activate the full healing capabilities of the substance. Until this happens individuals are not truly considered *ngangkari*, even if they possess a sufficient amount of *nguwa*.

The physical effects of *nguwa* during the maturation process are the primary reason children *ngangkari* often lose their powers as they grow older. Full healing abilities can harm children and, as a consequence, these powers are generally not released until after initiation. The frequent illness caused by *nguwa* is also much more difficult for a child like Alan to bear. He would have to endure the sicknesses caused by his *nguwa* for over a decade before he could be opened up. Consequently, Margaret regularly urged George to remove the child's *nguwa*. A few months later when Alan was still suffering the effects of the *nguwa*, George placed the substance back inside his own body. He said, "That baby needs to be healthy like other babies.'

Although some men, such as Jacob, had possessed *nguwa* for most of their adult lives, it was not uncommon for individuals like Alan and George to obtain, and then lose, the substance. While men wished to preserve their *nguwa*, for many, being a *ngangkari* was temporary. Not only could *nguwa* be removed by other individuals, it could also be destroyed. This occurs when *nguwa* becomes too hot, usually the result of prolonged illness or consuming hot foods, such as chilies, tea, or alcohol.[7] George partially attributed the disappearance of his *ngawa* years ago to his habit of pouring large amounts of Tabasco® sauce on his meals—a habit he was careful to alter once he regained *nguwa*. In addition to spicy cuisine or foods consumed at a high temperature, any food that noticeably increased body temperature was considered a risk. Residents of Lajamanu stated that the food most responsible for the loss of *nguwa* was alcohol. A number of former *ngangkari* reported permanently losing their abilities as a result of frequent drinking. Several years ago, George stated that he was particularly concerned for Carl and Donald, who often travelled to Katherine or Alice Springs and drank to excess.

While Lajamanu is a dry community—the possession or consumption of alcohol within ten miles has been prohibited since 1979—some individuals, particularly young men, consume alcohol on a regular basis and in large quantities.[8] One resident said, "*Yapa*, they have to drink a lot. One can, not enough, two cans, not enough, three cans, not enough. We have to drink until we get drunk. *Kardiya*, they can have only one beer. Not this mob [Aboriginal people]." While alcohol abuse is acknowledged as contributing to a variety of health problems—including accidental death, kidney failure, and liver disease—in Lajamanu, excessive drinking was also believed to injure the spiritual self, irreparably harming both *nguwa* and the *pirlirrpa*. One man explained that because the *pirlirrpa* is anchored in the kidneys and alcoholism can result in kidney failure, the *pirlirrpa* could also be debilitated and destroyed by alcohol. In addition, the heat of intoxication caused *nguwa* to become ineffective and slowly fade away. When drunk, *ngangkari* were unable to diagnose and heal. If these episodes occurred frequently and for extended periods, a *ngangkari* could lose his *nguwa* completely. Furthermore, intoxicated *ngangkari*, with their senses dulled and powers weakened, were especially unable to protect their *nguwa* against sober healers seeking to increase their abilities.

In addition to foods and beverages, illness was also considered to produce heat, which could lead to the weakening and loss of *nguwa*. A Warlpiri woman commented, "*Nguwa* can't stay in a sick body." I was often told of how the heat of a *yarda* caused a *ngangkari* to be temporarily divested of his abilities. If left untreated, a spiritual illness could result in the permanent loss of *nguwa*. While magical pathogens are one cause, so is chronic physical illness. On a recent visit, I found myself sitting under a bough-shelter with Jacob. As we were talking, Jacob removed his shoe, pointing to where three toes had been amputated as a result of diabetes complications. Jacob remarked that after the operation, he noticed that his healing abilities had decreased. He implicated diabetes for this loss. He asked, "How can you heal when you are sick all the time?"

When I first arrived in Lajamanu, men who had lost *nguwa*, like George, mourned its absence but believed that they could in time regain the substance either from nature or another individual. A particular piece of *nguwa* could be destroyed but a time could come when it would be replaced. Today, this has changed. The number of *ngangkari* has significantly declined. Jacob is now one of the few *ngangkari* left in the community. Individuals that were treating spiritual illness only a few years ago now report that their abilities are severely weakened, as with Jacob, or have disappeared altogether, as with Carl and Donald. Like many others in the community, Jacob blamed the high rates of chronic illness and alcohol abuse, which are in turn considered the result of colonialism and continued government management. Given that these conditions showed no signs of abating, Jacob speculated that a time would come when there were no longer *ngangkari* living in Lajamanu. Then, opening his wallet, Jacob produced his "Basic Card." As many Aboriginal individuals receiving welfare payments had the majority of their monies placed in managed accounts from which cash could not be withdrawn, these cards allowed them to make purchases at the shop. Jacob added, "We have nothing. They take it all."

While *nguwa* is a magical substance that bestows healing abilities, it is also a locus through which the conditions of life in Lajamanu are expressed. As the previous chapter demonstrated, non-Aboriginal foods are regularly blamed for high rates of Aboriginal illness. In this instance, chronic illness and alcohol abuse threaten not only physical health but also spiritual well-being. In Jacob's case, his diabetes resulted in the loss of toes and *nguwa*. Chronic ill health, the demise of *ngangkari*, and continued government interference are inextricably linked. Notions of *ngangkari* and *nguwa* reflect social and political perspectives borne out of contemporary struggles within Aboriginal communities. The conditions of life in Lajamanu—family relations, demand sharing, alcohol abuse, government interventions, and chronic illness—are articulated through Warlpiri cosmology.

Sorcerers

Like notions of *pirlirrpa* and *nguwa*, sorcery and sorcery accusations are situated firmly within the social context of Lajamanu. Historically, anthropologists have viewed narratives regarding sorcery as an expression of social relations between Aboriginal individuals or families (Reid 1983).[9] In Lajamanu, sorcerers or *jarnpa* are males that use sacred, secret magic to injure and kill others. A man is taught the songs and ceremonies by senior male relatives as he is initiated into ever-higher levels of understanding. Although I have met men who have hinted that they perhaps possessed such knowledge, its actual use was never confirmed. Given that the rituals required to ensorcell another individual is sacred, secret, and restricted to senior men, detailed information is never revealed to non-initiates. Furthermore, confessing to the practice of sorcery would mark an individual as a murderer or attempted murderer, resulting in retribution from the community and those targeted. Consequently, while I have been told many tales, I have never met a self-proclaimed *jarnpa*.

In an effort to escape detection and hide their identities, *jarnpa* are thought to be capable of performing sorcery that is not only deadly but also cunning, such as stealing souls and creating zombie-like beings.[10] "Strong" *jarnpa* are able to sing the *pirlirrpa* out of the body and imprison it in a small container, which is then hidden underground or behind an inconspicuous object in the bush. While imprisoned, the *pirlirrpa* cries for its body. Deprived of its life force, the physical self rapidly decays, mental faculties disappear, and death becomes inevitable. Without the aid of a *ngangkari* to locate and restore the trapped *pirlirrpa*, the victim's soul will remain hidden, eternally crying out for a body that has perished. *Jarnpa* also use techniques to avoid being blamed for a death. Referred to as *jajinjinpa*, a sorcerer is capable of killing a man and then reanimating his corpse. Seeing the victim walking around, community residents assume he is healthy and alive. Under the control of the *jarnpa*, the victim starts an unprovoked fight with a kinsman or bystander. The slightest blow then causes the victim's body to fall down dead. Consequently, the kinsman or bystander is found guilty of murder, not the *jarnpa*.

Given the clandestine nature of *jarnpa*, most people tend to make sorcery accusations based upon interpersonal relations. I have been told of sorcery prompted by disputes over women, access to cash, rights to land, and Australian football games. While watching an important football match between Lajamanu and its rival, Yuendumu, a player sustained a severe fall and was unable to move off the field unassisted. I was told later that a *yarda* had been sung under the field to prevent the team from winning.

The activities of *jarnpa* can also be revealed through dreams.[11] After experiencing symptoms for weeks, Sarah reported a dream in which she saw Virgil, her former father-in-law, approach an unidentified group of men sitting around a fire. Virgil handed money to one of the men, asking him to sing Sarah. The following morning, Sarah's mother, Deborah, claimed to have had an identical dream. While Sarah obtained treatment from *ngangkari*, both women began publically accusing Virgil of causing of Sarah's suffering. Other women told me that, given Virgil's relationship with Sarah, it was not surprising that he would wish to cause her harm. Eleven months earlier Sarah's husband had become drunk and severely beat her and her two children. While she was in the hospital recovering, Virgil threatened to kill Sarah if his son was arrested. Sarah claimed that she told the police not to prosecute but Virgil's son was nevertheless imprisoned. One woman stated that by ensorcelling Sarah, Virgil was getting revenge for his son's incarceration.

Firmly embedded in the everyday world of sports ovals, police reports, hospitals, and prisons, accusations of sorcery clearly articulate social relations. While the first example was motivated by team rivalry, the second reflects gender relations in Lajamanu. Sarah's accusation gives voice to her own vulnerability as a woman living in a community with a high rate of domestic violence. By focusing on sorcery—a skill belonging only to men—and accusing Virgil, his son, the sorcerer, and those around the circle that allowed the transaction to take place, Sarah is highlighting men's role in women's suffering. Furthermore, Sarah's narrative stresses her inability to stop the legal proceedings against her husband. Portrayed as powerless in the face of the criminal justice system, Sarah shifts the responsibility for her husband's imprisonment from herself to the state.

Sarah's accusation of Virgil is but one example of a sorcery narrative. Age, gender, marital status, income, and family history all impact the way in which individuals configure their relationships vis-à-vis others. Ultimately this diversity is reflected in tales of sorcery. For instance, older men linked settlement with sorcery and high mortality rates.[12] They blamed crowded conditions around ration stations and in communities for causing violent disputes to erupt more frequently, leading those involved to employ sorcery. One senior man related, "There were many fights and one man would sing another. Many people died. But now those men are gone." Older residents of Lajamanu commented that these deaths, coupled with a lack of interest by young men, meant that the number of *jarnpa* in the community was steadily declining. One old man said, "The young fellas don't know anything. They watch TV instead of learning songs." In contrast, younger individuals focused on contemporary struggles over money, women, and resources. In many cases, sorcery attacks implicate the alleged sorcerer's close kin as well as that of the victim. Invoking relationships in a very public manner, retribution can embroil family members in long-running disputes and conflicts. Sorcery accusations "entail the reification of kinship relations" (Schwarz 2010b, 63).

Sorcery allegations like Sarah's are invariably debated and contested throughout the community. These narratives are dialogues rather than monologues. In the case of Sarah's illness, Larry, a senior man, strongly disagreed with the hypothesis that Sarah had been ensorcelled by Virgil. He contended that Sarah was not suffering from a spiritual illness at all; she had inherited a heart disease from her mother, Deborah. Larry emphasized that it was a scientific fact that some illnesses are inherited. He explained, "Her genes are bad. That is why she is sick. It is her mother's fault because she gave rubbish genes." Larry remarked that it was no surprise Sarah was unwell now as she was always suffering from illness episodes. Larry was well aware of her frequent visits to hospital and the rheumatic heart fever she had contracted as a child. As we talked, the conversation shifted from Sarah's illness to Deborah's recent decision to quit her job at the clinic to work exclusively at the Women's Centre.

Larry stated that Deborah had caused "trouble" and "turned her back on the community." He added that although Deborah claimed her departure from the clinic was a result of high work stress, this was not an acceptable excuse. Larry felt she should resume her job as an Aboriginal Health Worker immediately. Returning to the topic of Sarah's illness, Larry stressed that sorcery was not the correct diagnosis. He believed she should be seeing heart doctors at the Katherine hospital rather than *ngangkari* in Lajamanu.

Larry's rejoinder illustrates that sorcery is not the only way in which relationships are given voice. Far from relying exclusively on cosmologies of spirit beings or sorcerers, Lajamanu residents can use and manipulate biomedical explanations to disclose and comment upon social tensions in a way similar to sorcery accusations. Like Sarah's indictment of Virgil, Larry's statement also articulates gender concerns. With Deborah's departure from the clinic, treatment would be provided solely by non-Aboriginal female nurses. Already a socially difficult place for men to seek care, this situation was made worse without an Aboriginal Health Worker. While women could continue to benefit from Deborah's expertise at the Women's Centre, the men could not. Using a biomedical explanation that casts a woman as the cause, Larry absolves himself and other men from blame while simultaneously condemning Deborah's choice to resign from the clinic.

While sorcery can be a useful way to link illness and social relations, so can biomedicine and the language of science. The realms of sorcery and genetics are not as different as they might at first appear. Biomedical ideas are situated within local ontologies and deployed to reflect social concerns and ideas. Although sorcery accusations remain an idiom through which relations are expressed and negotiated, a conversation about the nutritional content of food or the etiology of heart disease is also capable of remarking upon the behavior of individuals or groups. In Lajamanu, biomedicine has been made local and integrated into cosmological beliefs and customary regulations.

Ghosts, Ancestral Sprits, and UFOs

Biomedicine is only one example of the ways in which contemporary dialogues invoke local cosmologies, kinship, and experience to comment critically upon social relations. Examining a tale of bulldozers driven by non-Aboriginal workers who allegedly unearthed a rainbow serpent,

Merlan (2005, 173) observed that, "Despite local perceptions and the objectively great degree of segregation of Aborigines in many aspects of daily life from whites, one is not justified in assuming radical boundedness between black and white 'worlds.'" Examining the intercultural illustrates the ways in which ontologies can be reconfigured and redeployed to highlight not only relationships between Warlpiri residents, as with Sarah's illness, but also tensions between Aboriginal and non-Aboriginal people. By invoking discourse that is recognized throughout Australia, such as biomedicine, local ideas are effectively communicated to a non-Aboriginal audience. Warlpiri people engage issues of race by uniting local cosmological themes—like belonging, trespass, and punishment—with global symbols. To illustrate this point, I will compare narratives of ghosts and ancestral spirits with those of UFOs.

In Lajamanu, the two most discussed spirit beings are *kuku* and *milalpa*. Upon death, the body's link to the *pirlirrpa* is permanently severed and corporeal life ceases. However, the spirit continues to exist, dividing into two aspects. The first—*milalpa* or the ancestral spirit—returns to the land from which it originated. The second—*kuku* or ghost—remains in the community and embodies the social aspect of the personality.[13] Invisible to everyone except *ngangkari*, *kuku* are the most publicly discussed spirit beings in Lajamanu. Because they frequent settled areas, *kuku* are said to regularly impact the lives of residents. Attracted to the people and objects of their former life, *kuku* roam through the community and the surrounding bush in the evening. Aggressive and malevolent, a *kuku* is likely to ensorcell anyone it accidentally encounters. To discourage visits by *kuku*, the names, belongings, and homes of recently deceased individuals are no longer used. At night, people walk in groups and speak in hushed tones. Despite these precautions, individuals are nevertheless ensorcelled by *kuku*. Though rarely fatal, being sung by a ghost can cause discomfort and suffering. In most cases, a *ngangkari* is able to remove any pathogens implanted by a *kuku*. As the opening anecdote illustrated, while Warlpiri people affirm the existence of *kuku*, adults nevertheless fabricate ghost stories to quiet noisy children. On many occasions, I witnessed parents pointing to a dark window falsely claiming to have seen *kuku*. I spoke to one man who went so far as to dress in a white sheet to scare his children. Like many beliefs in Lajamanu, *kuku* are treated as both a reality and a convenient tool to influence the behavior of others.

In contrast to *kuku*, *milalpa* are spirits that return to the ancestral land from which they originated. Only found in the bush, *milalpa* maintain the vitality of the land and guard against trespassing. At night, *milalpa* will emerge from the ground to inspect the surrounding countryside. Approaching campsites, *milalpa* can recognize the *pirlirrpa* of those present. Individuals acknowledged as kin and traditional owners are unharmed. All others face being ensorcelled as punishment for trespassing. Individuals from other communities were particularly fearful of *milalpa* when camping in the vicinity of Lajamanu. Even those that had resided in Lajamanu for years sometimes became nervous spending the night in the bush surrounding the community. On one occasion when returning from Yuendumu, we decided to camp only 100 kilometers from Lajamanu, in hopes of finding game. After choosing our site, an older *ngangkari* reported seeing a *milalpa*. One of the women present insisted that we continue driving to another location before making camp.

Milalpa are not the only type of being that inhabits traditional land and is capable of recognizing and harming trespassers. *Warnayarra*, often referred to as rainbow serpents in anthropological literature, also guard land (Buchler and Maddock 1978; Merlan 2000; Munn 1973; Radcliffe-Brown 1926; Rose 1992). Dwelling in water sources such as rivers, water holes, underground soaks, rain clouds, and seasonal creeks such as the one running beside the community, these giant multicolored snakes pervade the landscape. While children took great pleasure in frolicking in the creek during the wet season, parents warned that the resident *warnayarra* could kill young swimmers from other communities whom it did not recognize. If travelling away from the community, individuals were particularly conscious of *warnayarra*. While visiting a large salt lake, several men expressed fear of being punished by the *warnayarra* because they were not traditional owners. Even though the lakebed was dry, it was assumed that numerous *warnayarra* were living under the surface and capable of causing harm to trespassers. It is only in one's own country that an individual can feel safe from dangerous forces.

Affiliation through country can act as an objectification of kin networks and a record of social ties (Myers 1986, 128). In this way, country can be a source of identity, distinguishing differing claims to land but also connecting individuals through these bonds. For instance, the hazards associated with visiting foreign land can be mitigated when a traditional owner and sponsor introduces a stranger to country. This act bestows protection upon the guest, which beings such as *milalpa* and *warnayarra* honor. Often when I spent the night camped in the bush, a senior man would sing to the *milalpa*, usually in the early evening, instructing them not to harm me. I was also introduced to *warnayarra* on a number of occasions while visiting rock pools. In each instance, a senior man, who was the acknowledged owner of the site, placed a small amount of water on my head while telling the *warnayarra* that I should not be injured. As Myers notes (1986, 151) among the Pintupi, the act of bestowing protection also acknowledges the dependency that a visitor has on his or her sponsor. Through beings such as *milalpa*, rights to country are politically asserted and legitimized.

While discussions of *kuku*, *milalpa*, and *warnayarra* permeated Aboriginal conversations in Lajamanu, non-Aboriginal residents generally had little or no knowledge of these beings or the dangers that they posed to trespassers. Nevertheless, similar narratives of belonging, protection, and traditional ownership were used in another context—one in which non-Aboriginal people did participate—UFOs. Soon after arriving in Lajamanu I discovered that conversations between Aboriginal and non-Aboriginal residents regarding extraterrestrials and flying saucers were common. I eventually interviewed fifteen Warlpiri people and three non-Aboriginal people, who claimed to have personally sighted a UFO. I met many others who imparted detailed information regarding the activities of "the aliens." Regardless of whether or not community residents had sighted a UFO, believed in them, or discounted the existence of extraterrestrials altogether, they discussed the aliens on a regular basis.

Accounts of flying saucers and extraterrestrials resembled popularized notions of UFOs that are reflected in American television and film. Both Aboriginal and non-Aboriginal people agreed that UFOs were spaceships piloted by extraterrestrial beings. Furthermore, the aliens were said to occasionally abduct those they encountered driving on lonely roads late at night. But unlike American tales of extraterrestrials conducting medical experiments on humans before releasing them, Warlpiri people stated that abductees were never returned. Ronald, an Aboriginal council employee, recounted how Bill, a non-Aboriginal allied health service provider, visited the community for little over a day before driving back to town in the late afternoon. Four days later Bill had still not contacted the community council to inform them of his safe return to Katherine. Ronald claimed that both Bill's supervisor and the police had been notified but neither knew his whereabouts. Although Ronald had never encountered a UFO himself, he was certain that Bill had been abducted and would never be heard from again.

Despite tales of abductions, Warlpiri people did not feel that they were at risk. Ronald commented that he, as an Aboriginal man, was safe from alien abduction, whereas non-Aboriginal people were not. After recounting the details of his sighting, Mark asserted that while he was scared at the sight of the ship, he was not worried about being taken because the desert was his country. Asked if he was referring to a specific site or area, he replied that the aliens knew that Warlpiri people belonged in the Tanami Desert so they had nothing to fear. The same was said of the community. One man claimed that *yapa* would never be taken because the aliens had seen them "sit down" in the community for years. Another commented, "The aliens do nothing to us. But *kardiya*, maybe they are just travelling, maybe at night, and not thinking about anything then those aliens come and take them." While non-Aboriginal people were considered to be the sole victims of abduction, it was possible to avoid this fate. I was told that I could drive through the desert safely at night by having Warlpiri people in the car with me. Even if a UFO should appear, it was believed that *kardiya* would not be taken as long as an Aboriginal person was present. It was only when non-Aboriginal people were travelling alone or with other non-Aboriginal people that they were in danger. I was told, "Don't worry. We will look after you." Once, when driving at night with a group of Aboriginal people to town, I was asked if I felt safe from the aliens. After replying that I wasn't sure, I was immediately told that my fellow passengers would protect me.

Taking a cue from popular media portrayals, Warlpiri narratives of UFO abductions echo themes of belonging, trespass, punishment, and protection that suffuse local cosmology, while also incorporating notions of race (Saethre 2007c). Just as *milalpa* are capable of recognizing individual owners of country, so are the aliens. Because non-Aboriginal people did not belong, they were in danger of abduction. Narratives of abductions mirrored those of punishment by ancestral forces for trespass. Furthermore, the manner in which protection was bestowed upon me in the bush resembles the way in which protection from abduction could also be obtained through the agency of Aboriginal people. But unlike narratives regarding *warnayarra*, which distinguish traditional owners by their family, site of conception, or their place of residence, abduction tales focus exclusively on race. The pervasive division in the community between *kardiya* and *yapa* that encompasses social networks, spaces, resources, technologies, education, traditions, and healing options was also a fundamental feature in UFO narratives. The only identity that the aliens seem to functionally acknowledge in humans was that of Aboriginal and non-Aboriginal.

Abduction narratives not only emphasize racial affiliation, they also delineate the relationship between these two groups. As non-Aboriginal people are incorporated into Warlpiri models of belonging through public discussions of sightings and abductions, relationships between Indigenous and non-Indigenous people are expressed. Integrating features of extraterrestrials with local cosmological themes, Warlpiri UFO tales provide an example through which the close encounters between Indigenous and non-Indigenous people can be understood. The actions of the aliens offer a powerful and unique validation of Aboriginality. Through elements of popular UFO stories, local cosmological themes, and the division between *yapa* and *kardiya*, alien abduction narratives are able to present an Aboriginal identity that is differentiated from non-Aboriginal identity and linked to belonging and continued ownership of land. Abductions affirm that Aboriginal people are at home and make a home in Lajamanu and the Tanami Desert in a way that non-Aboriginal people do not. Aliens demonstrate Warlpiri security, assurance, and belonging while highlighting non-Aboriginal foreignness and vulnerability.

Although often considered to be immune from the intervention of sorcery, non-Aboriginal people are victims of abductions. Furthermore, stories of UFOs incorporated non-Aboriginal people as both a subject and as an audience in a way that accounts of *milalpa* and *warnayarra* generally did not. Warnings of UFO abductions, including that of Bill's disappearance, were often conveyed to non-Aboriginal residents of the community. I was told, "You *kardiya* have to be careful because the aliens might get you." Ian, a medical researcher who spent only three months in the community, stated that he had been cautioned repeatedly about the risk of alien abduction. Many non-Aboriginal residents were initially skeptical; however, after spending longer periods of time living in the community, some began to re-evaluate their earlier disbelief. After residing in Lajamanu for over a year and having heard a number of stories regarding UFOs from Aboriginal people, a non-Aboriginal teacher confessed to gradually becoming more hesitant to drive long distances at night during the wet season, when most abductions were thought to occur. I believe a parallel can be made between tales of abductions and tales of *kuku*. *Kuku* are considered a real cause of illness as well as a device to make children behave. Similarly, UFOs are seen and experienced while also acting as a cautionary story for non-Aboriginal workers.

More than just an admonition, tales of abductions also reflect the very real mobility and impermanence of most non-Aboriginal residents. For instance, Bill's abduction is illustrative of the current state of medical service provision in many remote Aboriginal communities, where allied health workers provided services on a brief and sporadic basis (Heil 2006, 106; Lea 2008, 57). Like other health care professionals, Bill visited the community for a very short period of time and left, never to be heard from again. While other non-Aboriginal residents worked and lived in the community for longer periods, none believed that it would be a permanent home. After a few months or years, non-Aboriginal workers departed the community, often never to return. Stories of Aboriginal abductions portray the tendency of non-Aboriginal residents to metaphorically vanish from Lajamanu.

Like discussions of saturated fat or genetics, UFOs create a sort of parity between Aboriginal and non-Aboriginal (Saethre 2007a). Similarly, the rainbow serpent has also been transformed into a creator spirit within a single unified Indigenous theology (McDonald 2010, 57). One result of the colonial encounter in Australia is that "Indigenous knowledge is no longer self-evident; it must be assessed relative to the knowledge of the colonizers, if it is not to be abandoned as worthless, it must either be consigned to a separate domain or made commensurate with the knowledge of the other through some kinds of articulation" (Beckett 1993, 691). Warlpiri ideas of the world are incorporated into and "made commensurate" with both national and international narratives through dialogues such as Ronald's description of Bill's abduction, Larry's statement that Sarah was suffering from a genetic condition inherited from her mother, Jacob's tale of losing *nguwa* after an amputation precipitated by diabetes complications, and Ethan's assertion that too much alcohol can damage the *pirlirrpa*. Consequently, Indigenous cosmologies are not isolated domains. Rather, they fit within and reflect contemporary social settings that include biomedical discourse, chronic illness, and racial inequality, while simultaneously acting as a powerful narrative to express and contest personal and collective viewpoints.

CHAPTER 4

Medical Systems and Illness Experience

D espite the almost ubiquitous presence of biomedicine around the globe, a great deal of treatment occurs outside of clinical confines. Indigenous practices are invariably contrasted with those of biomedicine. In the extensive literature that exists, the former is characterized as traditional and grounded in cultural beliefs, while the latter is considered scientific. As a result, medical beliefs and treatments are often conceptualized in terms of medical systems—internally coherent structures of meaning that encompass ideas, treatments, technologies, and values (Janzen 1978; Press 1980). Cast as the product of cultural difference, Indigenous medical systems are commonly portrayed as static and homogenous within a medical context (Kleinman and Benson 2006b, 835). Furthermore, Indigenous beliefs and practices are generally viewed as limiting, rather than encouraging, health outcomes (Gordon 1988; Taylor 2007). Through medical narratives, Indigeneity becomes essentialized, reified, and cast as fundamentally different from, and at odds with, clinical treatment.

This is particularly evident in Australia where researchers, medical professionals, and health advocates often assume that two contrasting and incommensurate medical systems exist: Aboriginal and biomedical. Aboriginal healing beliefs are widely characterized as concerned about the social health of the group, while biomedicine is thought to concentrate on the biological individual (Mobbs 1991; Nathan and Leichleitner 1983). Portrayed as reductionist and impersonal, clinical treatment is cast as focusing solely on physical and environmental factors (Devanesen 1985, 33; Morgan, Slade, and Morgan 1997, 589). As a result, Aboriginal and biomedical systems are believed to be "vastly different in philosophy and practice" (Nathan and Leichleitner 1983, 72), and are compared in terms of a "stark contrast" (Mobbs 1991, 302) or "cultural gap" (Eastwell 1973, 1012). "Competing" (Nathan and Leichleitner 1983, 70), "poor compatibility" (Maher 1999, 234) and "clash" (Sutton 2005, 1) are common ways of characterizing the relationship between the two medical approaches. These differences are widely believed to create barriers to effective biomedical care (Heil 2006; Mobbs 1991; Public Accounts Committee 1996; Saggers and Gray 1991).

The division between allopathic and Aboriginal medicine with respect to ideas about illness and healing is not confined to health researchers and medical professionals. It is one that Aboriginal people themselves widely recognize (Maher 1999, 234; Nathan and Leichleitner 1983, 133; Reid 1983, 134). During discussions with Warlpiri people, I was often told that two distinct medical traditions and treatment systems existed: *yapa-kurlangu* and *kardiya-kurlangu*. Residents asserted that the former included *ngangkari* and bush medicines, while the latter included biomedical techniques and technologies. Furthermore, I was informed that only *ngangkari* could treat a *yapa-kurlangu* disease, such as spiritual illness. Consequently, it appeared as if these two healing options were discrete. In practice, however, I found this was not the case.

While many statements focusing on illness beliefs made by Lajamanu residents highlighted and contrasted the differences between Aboriginal and non-Aboriginal etiologies and therapies, the practical way in which people sought care for a specific illness was far more integrated. I discovered that individuals concurrently employed numerous healing aids and technologies, a trend that has been—and continues to be—widely documented (Beck 1985, 84; Cawte 1974, 43; Cutter 1976, 38; Devitt and McMasters 1998; Dussart 2009; Gray 1979, 172; Skov 1994, 20; Tonkinson 1982, 229). Similar to narratives surrounding hunting and gathering, I came to notice that generalized statements did not always hold true in practice. Diagnoses often changed, as did treatment choice. Despite declarations stressing the incommensurability of *kardiya* and *yapa* techniques, a variety of treatments were utilized without a clash. Consequently, I believe the assumption that biomedicine and Indigenous healing beliefs are invariably conflicting and incompatible needs to be re-evaluated. Notions of distinct medical systems seem to reproduce perceptions of ethnic and racial identity rather than accurately reflecting the everyday reality of treatment behavior.

Statements touting the discord between Indigenous and biomedical systems tend to disregard that illness is both an experience and an idiom. On one hand, it is lived—uncertainty, stress, discomfort, and pain often suffuse the experience of illness. On the other hand, narratives of illness provide an interpretation of the natural and social world. When researching Indigenous responses to ill health, a great deal of attention has centered on the idiom, whereas the day-to-day experience of disease is often overlooked. There has been a tendency to draw conclusions based almost exclusively on notional representations such as those that are expressed in interviews or verbal interactions. Nathan and Leichleitner (1983, 132) state, "What has been recorded is what people said occurs and not what may happen in actual practice. Nevertheless, it is a sociological truism that beliefs dictate actions." I disagree. In Lajamanu, illness experience also motivated action and, at times, these actions could appear to contradict statements of belief. Consequently, it is important to situate responses to disease within everyday life, rather than accepting models that "compare societies not in terms of empirical realities but in terms of reified concepts" (Jackson 1989, 11).

To illustrate the ways in which a variety of treatment methods are practically utilized by Indigenous people, I will explore the events surrounding one of George's illness episodes. After experiencing symptoms for three weeks before being evacuated to Katherine Hospital, his sickness was variously attributed to a mild case of the flu, sorcery from an unknown individual, and heart failure. George sought assistance from a number of individuals including family members, several *ngangkari*, two female nurses, and myself. While *ngangkari* magically removed sharpened bones, poisoned blood, and other pathogens from his body, doctors and nurses prescribed pharmaceuticals, blood pressure checks, and EKGs. I supplied George with vitamin C. By the end of his illness episode George had used healing options that were considered to be biomedical and Aboriginal in much the same way.

Diagnoses and Treatments

George first noticed he was ill while visiting Yuendumu, a Warlpiri community approximately 600 kilometers south of Lajamanu. Feeling lethargic as well as experiencing a low fever and stomach cramps, George believed he was suffering from *minta*. Although popularly translated as the flu, *minta* is a distinct category of physical disease. Believed to be caused by a wide variety of natural events, such as contact with an infected person, malnutrition, cold weather, excessive alcohol, or poor hygiene, the symptoms of *minta* often include fever, chills, aches, and diarrhea. A case of *minta* could be considered the result of a virus going around the community, passed from one person to the next through physical contact. Alternatively, abnormal temperature variations in the body, for instance becoming too cold during the winter or too hot after excessive drinking, could be blamed. Spoiled, excessively fatty *kardiya-kurlangu* meat, unfamiliar food, or poorly treated water is also thought to precipitate *minta*. As George's symptoms appeared soon after his arrival in Yuendumu, he believed the illness was triggered by drinking the community's mineralized water.

Although he was feeling ill, George did not to attend the clinic. *Minta* is a frequent fact of life in Lajamanu and many suffers choose to treat the symptoms themselves. Suffering from *minta* as much as three times a month, George regularly carried a bottle of paracetamol in his pocket. While the causes of *minta* may vary from episode to episode, the common curatives remain the same: resting, consuming liquids, and using both biomedical and bush medicines. Because *minta* causes the body to become unusually cold, sufferers will often sleep by a fire or warm place to correct this imbalance. In addition, George also consumed spicy food to restore his body's heat but was careful not to eat too much lest he lose his *nguwa*. After he fell ill in Yuendumu, George reported taking paracetamol and resting. He said that he would have preferred to use bush medicines but stated that he was not feeling well enough to gather the necessary herbs. Like many residents, George praised bush medicines but seldom used them. When initially asked about his illness, George replied, "This is normal for me. I don't have bad health. *Minta* just goes around a lot." Although he considered himself to be fit, George was obese, suffered from hypertension, and seldom engaged in any exercise.

Three days passed and George's health continued to decline. No longer feeling well enough to drive home, he remained in Yuendumu. Given the persistence of symptoms despite his self-medication, George began to question his initial diagnosis. He suspected that his illness could be spiritual rather than physical. Consequently, four days after the onset of symptoms, he consulted a *ngangkari*, who discovered and removed a *yarda* implanted inside George's body. Although a tangible bone was not displayed after the treatment, George reported feeling confident that his health would improve. After two days, his symptoms began to subside. George returned to the *ngangkari* and, after another examination, was assured that the previous treatment was indeed effective. Having received a clean bill of health, George drove home. Spending only two days in

Lajamanu, George traveled north to Katherine, where his symptoms returned: a low fever, stomach cramps, and now joint aches. Because the extraction of a *yarda* can temporarily debilitate the physical body, George initially speculated that he had contracted *minta*. But after additional deliberation, George concluded that his symptoms indicated the continuing presence of a *yarda*. Either the *ngangkari* in Yuendumu had failed to detect an additional pathogen or the original *yarda* had magically returned. George, once again too ill to return home, consulted a *ngangkari* in Katherine. His suspicions were confirmed when a *yarda* was found and removed. After a few days of rest, George once again felt well enough to drive back to Lajamanu.

George, like many Warlpiri people with whom I spoke, associated a wide variety of symptoms with spiritual illness. Headaches, bodily pains, nausea, fever, and vomiting could all indicate the presence of a spiritual illness. However, these symptoms are similar to those of physical illness. In many instances, individuals cannot diagnose spiritual illness based only upon the symptoms. Often a dream, recent experience with supernatural beings, or the verdict of a *ngangkari* are marshaled as collaborating evidence. As symptoms can change, dreams can be contradictory, and differing *ngangkari* can give differing opinions, a diagnosis of spiritual illness is debated, affirmed, or contested based on what are seen to be the most relevant circumstances. Consequently, spiritual illness is not simply a discrete set of bodily sensations; it is a social state.

Upon his return to Lajamanu, George confessed that he had no idea who had implanted the *yarda* in his body. Perhaps, George mused, he had accidentally walked in front of a *yarda* meant for someone in Yuendumu. Perhaps it was caused by a strong ghost looking to do someone harm. In any case, George did not believe that the *yarda* was the result of a personal attack motivated by hatred or that his health was critically threatened. Although he continued to experience mild symptoms, George was certain that he would make a full recovery. Despite George's confidence that the treatments he had received were efficacious, his wife, Margaret, had doubts. As George recounted tales of his treatments in Yuendumu and Katherine, Margaret remained silent. Disagreeing with his diagnosis, she believed that George was suffering from an acute case of *minta*. Margaret stated that seeing a *ngangkari* was helpful in some cases but not in this one. She was sure that her husband was suffering from a physical complaint and therefore, should attend the clinic. Urging George to consult the nurses, Margaret stressed that prescription pharmaceuticals were the best method of treatment given his symptoms. She worried that without biomedical intervention his illness could become severe, perhaps even developing into pneumonia.

George, however, did not concur with his wife's assessment. He said, "I am sick *yapa* way. Only strong *ngangkari* man can cure me. That is our culture, our way." George repeatedly referred to his illness as spiritual, stating that he would not consult the nursing staff because they were only effective at treating physical complaints such as diabetes or *minta.* Like George, Warlpiri people affirmed that despite a wealth of biomedical technology, the clinic was unable to recognize or treat spiritual illness, such as that caused by sorcery. Liddy said, "Those doctors, they don't understand Aboriginal sickness. They do x-rays but they still can't see that bone inside." In contrast, diabetics asserted that *ngangkari* were unable to treat their illness. Consequently, Lajamanu residents asserted that treatment choice was determined by the category of disease, spiritual or physical. Bill said, "Maybe if you have *minta* those nurses can make you right. But there are some things that they can't fix. You have to be sure which one you have."

Listening to these statements gives the impression that Warlpiri people follow a clearly demarcated and unambiguous treatment regimen depending on the cause of the illness: biomedicine for physical illness and *ngangkari* for spiritual illness.[1] If this is the case, then diagnosis and etiological beliefs become two very important issues in determining care. A conviction that an illness is caused by sorcery could delay or even prohibit a visit to the clinic, which, if the illness were serious, could lead to death. Hence, some health researchers and medical professionals view the belief in sorcery as fundamentally detrimental to the clinical care of Aboriginal people. Sutton (2005, 9) remarks, "One of the more powerful traditional factors in preventing adaptation to contemporary conditions is the instilling in many Aboriginal people, from an early age, of a causal theory in which most serious illnesses and most deaths are due to the ill-will and sorcery of other people." This view seems to be based on two assumptions. The first is that Aboriginal and biomedical systems are mutually exclusive. Employing the diagnoses and therapies of one automatically precludes the use of the other. The second assumption is that diagnosis is the foremost factor influencing illness behavior. These two assumptions may at first appear reasonable given the views of researchers examined at the beginning of the chapter and those of Warlpiri people above. However, before accepting these conclusions, it is necessary to examine the actions of individuals, such as George, during actual illness episodes.

Ngangkari and Pharmaceuticals

Twelve days after the onset of symptoms in Yuendumu, George's health continued to deteriorate. Hoping to locate "stronger" *ngangkari*, he decided to seek treatment in Daguragu, a Gurindji community 100 kilometers to the north. Suffering from intermittent fevers and feeling too ill to make the trip alone, George was accompanied by his wife and children. Over the next ten days, George repeatedly consulted *ngangkari* who magically extracted a number of pathogens from his body. Once again feeling that his symptoms were subsiding and convinced that a complete recovery was eminent, George returned to Lajamanu. As had occurred after his trip to Katherine, George told stories of his sessions with *ngangkari*. In addition to *yarda*, a number of other objects were found in his body. When a *ngangkari* produced a hairstring after one consultation, George admitted he was both surprised and impressed. On another occasion, a *ngangkari* made an invisible incision and sucked out dirty blood from his body. Although George had not completely recuperated, he did not doubt the efficacy of the powerful healing techniques he had experienced.

Unfortunately, George's health declined again only a few days after his homecoming. As time passed, his body seemed to swell in size. Once more, George regularly sought treatment from *ngangkari*. Almost every afternoon, he could be seen driving around the community requesting care. On a single day, George could have several *yarda* removed. After one treatment session, George reported that an entire dillybag (a small sack used to carry objects) was pulled from his body. This, he said, was the reason the pathogens could not be effectively banished: when a dillybag is magically implanted into a victim, it is able to regenerate *yarda*. Although the removal of the dillybag buoyed his spirits for a few days, George's health continued to deteriorate. Except for a few brief periods, it was clear that his illness was not dissipating, despite assurances that the *yarda*, blood, hairstring, or dillybag had been eliminated.

While George continued to visit *ngangkari*, the female members of his family pressured him to attend the clinic. His wife and daughter claimed that the treatments provided by the *ngangkari* would never be effective. Margaret said, "Sometimes *ngangkari* are [good] but not now. He thinks it is *yarda* but it isn't. Probably there is something wrong with his organs, and those sisters could find out." Margaret stated that the only way he could be healed was by attending the clinic. Several other female family members also urged him to seek biomedical care but George remained resistant to consulting the nurses. He repeated that his illness was of a spiritual nature and any attempt at clinical treatment would be ineffective. George told me, "The sisters can't do anything to make me [good]. I have a spiritual illness."

Although his continued refusals to attend the clinic were based on the assertion that his illness was spiritual, George nevertheless sought treatments considered appropriate for physical disease. After returning from Daguragu, he came to my home requesting vitamin C tablets, which he had begun taking months earlier to treat *minta*. As I gave George the vitamin C, he commented that he would have preferred to take bush medicines in addition to the vitamins. George reiterated that *yapa-kurlangu* therapies, like bush medicines and *ngangkari*, were often more effective than *kardiya-kurlangu* alternatives. Nevertheless, he stated that vitamins, like bush medicine, were "natural."

Two days later, George again came to my door seeking remedies. On this occasion, he requested prescription medication. George explained that despite taking a steady supply of paracetamol since the onset of his illness, it was doing little to control his fevers and discomfort. Mentioning that several months earlier he was prescribed pills that were significantly more effective, George asked if I had either these pills or an equivalent. When pressed for more information, George could only tell me that a male nurse had given him the medication for a high fever. In addition to an analgesic, George also requested antibiotics, which he believed would reduce the swelling throughout his body and allow him to breathe easier. When I explained that I did not have either of these items, George suggested that I could get them for him at the clinic. He noted that as a result of my extended research, I had a relationship with the nursing staff. Replying that I did not believe that the nurses would honor my requests for prescription medication until they examined him, I offered to accompany George to the clinic. He refused.

Given the disparity between George's assertions that biomedicine could not treat a spiritual illness and his requests for pharmaceuticals, it is apparent that the actions of Warlpiri people are more complex than many of their statements indicate. When examining the practical tactics that individuals use to alleviate suffering, researchers have noted that

"Explaining the tenacity of traditional beliefs and expectations in terms of the meaning system of the community does not help to clarify why non-Western people typically make heavy use of the Western medical system" (Welsch 1991, 35). Lajamanu residents are accustomed to taking pills when they feel ill—regardless of whether the disease is thought to be physical or spiritual—despite stating that *kardiya-kurlangu* medicines were less effective than *yapa-kurlangu* ones. Narratives regarding models of diagnosis and treatment instantiate representations of the social world, but actual treatment behavior is structured by the practical utilization of this social world.

Social relations, personal connections, and gender concerns play important roles in determining treatment. Of the *ngangkari* that George consulted, all but one was immediate family, close classificatory kin, or senior men that had ties to him through ceremony. Many people prefer to consult *ngangkari* within close social circles because of the trust and obligations these relationships entail. Furthermore, residents often base their opinion of a *ngangkari* on their relationship with that person. Howard said, "I don't believe in *ngangkari*. They are all fake, except my uncle. He is a real *ngangkari*." If a *ngangkari* is unknown and there is not a trusted individual to vouch for him, his very status as a healer may be questioned. While cosmology provides the groundwork of belief about illness, it is made manifest through a personal knowledge and trust of the individual providing treatment.

In contrast to *ngangkari*, George did not have strong relationships with the nursing staff in the clinic. Few nurses stayed in Lajamanu long enough to build rapport with its inhabitants. Of the many nurses that I interviewed, fourteen months was the longest period any had spent working in Lajamanu. Once a nurse departed, it was often difficult to find a replacement. To fill the gap, a string of temporary staff, some serving less than two weeks before being replaced by another temporary nurse, were employed. In the past, George only had brief interactions with the current nurses, Tina and Dorothy. The importance of having personal knowledge of treatment providers and its impact on the health-seeking behavior of Aboriginal people are well-known among health care professionals and researchers. A desire to encourage connections with the clinic and thereby raise consultation rates was one of the primary objectives of the Aboriginal Health Worker Program (Devanesen 1982, 21; Josif and Elderton 1992, 11; Willis 1985, 31). It was also a factor prompting concern over the high turnover of nursing staff in the Northern Territory (Cramer 1995, 23; Public Accounts Committee 1996, 52; Tatz 1972, 17).

Even if nurses worked for extended periods in Lajamanu, George would still have difficulty establishing relationships with them due to pervasive gender norms that play a central role in the utilization of clinical treatment options. Gender divisions exist throughout a wide range of Warlpiri activities, ceremonies, and locations (Dussart 2000; Meggitt 1962). Neither gender wishes to participate in activities or visit locations that are the domain of the other. If a breach occurs, the individual will often describe it as shameful, a concept which is much more severe than the English word suggests. Due to gender disparities in the medical profession, the vast majority of nurses were female. As a result, the clinic was considered to be a female space and was generally avoided by men.[2] One man explained his reluctance to seek treatment at the clinic for a gastrointestinal complaint, noting, "Too many [women]. It would be shame job." Men's disproportionate utilization of the clinic was reflected by an absence of medical charts: more than two-thirds belonged to women. When men did consult the nursing staff, they frequently chose to wait outside if a large number of women or those with whom they had avoidance relations were present. If a return visit to collect medication was needed, men often sent their wives.

Although George used diagnosis to justify his avoidance of the clinic, I believe social factors influenced his choice more than a belief that biomedicine would be ineffective. George's desire for pharmacopoeia indicated that he was not practically rejecting biomedical technology or *kardiya-kurlangu*, despite his statements to this effect. George was reluctant to enter a female space dominated by non-Aboriginal women. There is a marked difference between the utilization of biomedical treatment practitioners, which are predominantly non-Aboriginal female nurses, and biomedical treatments, including pills for headaches, cream for scabies, and insulin injections. While George sought to avoid the interactions entailed by the former, he nevertheless requested the latter. However, he did so through me, a male whom he had known for an extended period. A few months earlier, George had voluntarily presented for treatment at the clinic when a male nurse was on staff. I suspect that, had the nurse remained in Lajamanu, George would have been more likely to seek clinical treatment earlier in his illness episode. As a medical researcher noted, "I had a feeling that [Warlpiri people] had a great respect for some of the domains of Western medicine but their social context refrained them from exploiting them."

George's avoidance of the clinic should not be thought of as representative for all residents of Lajamanu. The importance of social factors in deciding treatment choice not only dissuaded some individuals from attending the clinic, it also encouraged others to consult nurses more than *ngangkari*. Women, particularly those with sick children, were more likely to present at the clinic than request the advice of a *ngangkari*. Despite suffering from slipped souls and other spiritual diseases, children were regularly taken to see the nursing staff as a matter of course. It was also possible for some individuals to build relationships with the nurses, often through repeated visits to the clinic or the presence of Aboriginal Health Workers. Sarah, whose mother had been employed as an Aboriginal Health Worker, was accustomed to visiting the clinic and stated that she often consulted the nurses when unsure of her health status.

While social relationships often influence initial treatment choice, other practitioners will be consulted if an illness episode continues. For instance, after an extended period of ill health, Sarah was diagnosed with systemic lupus erythematosus (SLE), a chronic inflammatory autoimmune disease that may, depending upon the individual case, be difficult to treat comprehensively. Initially, Sarah acknowledged that her illness was physical and agreed that the medical staff of the clinic were best equipped to treat her effectively. The nurses tried to control her symptoms with medication but Sarah reported that this did little good. Sarah continued to consult the clinic but the nurses began to feel that she was occupying an unreasonable amount of their time. Sarah was told repeatedly by the nursing staff that there was nothing else they could do for her; she was encouraged to stop coming to the clinic so often. A short time later, Sarah began consulting *ngangkari*.[3] As discussed in the previous chapter, after a revelatory dream Sarah believed that she was suffering from a spiritual disease, not a physical one. Asserting that she now knew the "real" cause of the illness, Sarah stopped attending the clinic regularly. Nevertheless, she still continued to take the pills given to her by the clinic on a sporadic basis as well as non-prescription medication, primarily paracetamol, which she purchased at the shop.

In an attempt to end the discomfort of disease, Lajamanu residents employ a variety of treatments—*ngangkari*, bush medicines, pharmaceuticals, and vitamins—without any perceived contradiction or conflict.

Wishing to curtail physical suffering, ill individuals will use whatever techniques or technologies are available. Not only do people use therapies simultaneously, social concerns appear to play a more critical role than idealized models. In examining treatment behavior in Papua New Guinea, Lewis (1993, 212) notes that, "Ordinarily, people are more concerned with efficacy and practical considerations than with explanatory consistency or logic." Despite statements stressing biomedicine's inability to treat sorcery, neither George nor Sarah expressed any unease about treating a spiritual illness with pharmaceuticals. Contrary to the earlier assertion by Nathan and Leichleitner (1983, 132), beliefs, or more precisely statements about beliefs, do not invariably dictate actions.

George's utilization of *ngangkari* and pharmaceuticals demonstrates that the two assumptions introduced earlier—(1) Aboriginal and biomedical systems are mutually exclusive and (2) diagnoses are the foremost factor influencing illness behavior—are false. Although notionally *ngangkari* and nurses are portrayed as discrete systems, George employed them in a similar manner. Whether having a *yarda* removed or requesting antibiotics, George obtained treatment from other males with whom he had relationships, while avoiding females with whom he did not. The day-to-day patterns of seeking care illustrate that people do not practically negotiate *yapa-kurlangu* or *kardiya-kurlangu* therapies in vastly different ways. Consequently, male avoidance of the clinic is actually an indication of the high degree to which biomedicine is integrated into the social fabric of Lajamanu.

The Clinic

Although gender norms might delay seeking treatment at the clinic, if symptoms become acute, almost everyone will consult the nurses. As the severity of an illness increases, social ease is eclipsed by a desire to become well. After becoming practically bedridden, George finally surrendered to his wife's pleas and agreed to go to the clinic. I would accompany him. Knowing that his medical condition was severe, George anticipated being evacuated to Katherine. Concerned that he would not receive the care of a *ngangkari* while hospitalized, George wanted to be examined one final time before presenting at the clinic. After having had a snake magically removed from his body the previous evening, George was keen to confirm that he was free of pathogens. But after a short drive around the community, it became apparent that we would not be able to find a *ngangkari* quickly. Rather than delay matters further, George broke off his search and drove to the clinic.[4]

After parking in front of the clinic, I helped George walk from the car to the front door. I noticed passers-by watching our progress. I knew it would not be long before his family and friends would arrive at the clinic concerned about his well-being. As we walked into the main room, one of the two nurses on staff that day, Tina, glanced up from a chart she was reading. Looking concerned, she instructed George to take a seat in the middle of the room and called for the second nurse, Dorothy. While Tina pulled up a blood pressure machine, Dorothy used a stethoscope to probe George's swollen chest for a heartbeat. His blood pressure was 218/196. George did not understand these numbers. While removing the apparatus Tina said in a brisk voice, "You are really sick. Do you understand? You should have come in sooner." Without another word, Tina and Dorothy walked across the room to confer quietly with one another. After a few moments, the nurses returned and announced that George would be evacuated to Katherine Hospital. Dorothy administered an injection while Tina rang for the medical plane.[5]

As we waited for the plane to arrive, George was led into an examination room to rest. Once he was settled in bed, Dorothy took me outside to discuss his condition. George, she said, was seriously ill. He appeared to be suffering from congestive heart failure. With his heart unable to pump blood as quickly or efficiently as needed, Dorothy speculated that George was probably retaining up to ten liters of extra fluid. His swollen appearance was the result of severe edema. We were soon joined by Tina, who added that George's heart could stop completely if he did not receive medical attention as soon as possible. Both nurses agreed that if George's heart arrested, they would not attempt to resuscitate him. His excessive weight would make it too difficult for them to accomplish on their own. They informed me that the clinic did not have adequate facilities or staff to cope with such an acute health crisis.

The nurses commented that George's condition was not a surprise. He had several risk factors for heart failure: high blood pressure, obesity, and lack of regular exercise. Further exacerbating matters, George repeatedly failed to pick up medication to control his hypertension. Tina recalled, "I told him months ago to take his medicine but he refused. I knew this would happen but what can you do? We can't force it down their throats." Both Tina and Dorothy expressed frustration that George had let his illness progress to such an advanced state. If he had come in weeks earlier, they said, he probably could have been treated in Lajamanu. Not only would this have prevented a considerable amount of suffering, it also would have saved the effort and expense of evacuating a medical emergency. Tina believed that, given his behavior and the severity of his condition, George would live for less than five years.

After the nurses excused themselves to fill out George's chart and complete the paperwork for his evacuation, I returned to his bedside. Soon Margaret arrived and we talked quietly with him. Tina briefly returned to check on George. She explained that his heart was "weak" and would collapse without immediate medical attention. Without another word, Tina left the room. She failed to mention either heart failure or edema and gave no indication of when George would be well enough to return to Lajamanu or what treatment awaited him in Katherine. George remained silent throughout Tina's explanation as he had for most of his examination. Although chided for not taking his medication regularly, he did not offer an excuse or confront the nurses. Margaret was so distressed she could only point to her own heart in silence. As the minutes passed, more and more members of the community came into the clinic to visit George.

While the nurses chatted in another room, the people sitting beside George began to discuss his symptoms. A consensus emerged that the fatigue, water retention, and nausea were caused not by a weak heart but by a snake. Many of those present commented that George was lucky that the snake had been removed the night before. The pain he was experiencing was probably just a residual side effect. Although a few people wanted George to be checked for additional pathogens, most believed that his symptoms would disappear in time without further assistance. An older man present commented that George could travel to Katherine with the confidence that the cause had been eliminated, thus ensuring a complete recovery. He said, "That snake was taken out. You will be fine now." Nevertheless, no one suggested that George remain in Lajamanu or refuse further medical care in Katherine.

Statements praising the abilities of local healers, such as those made at George's bedside, were not uncommon in Lajamanu. When medical facilities were utilized, it was often *ngangkari* that were ultimately credited with precipitating healing. For instance, after sustaining a sports injury, Jason was immediately taken to the clinic where he received treatment. After leaving the clinic, he consulted a *ngangkari*, who treated the injury as the result of sorcery perpetrated by the opposing team. Later, Jason stated that it was the *ngangkari*, not the nurses, who healed him. In the first chapter, Betty attributed her recovery to the removal of three *yarda*, not to the recent heart surgery that she had undergone. This trend has been recorded throughout the Northern Territory and Western Australia (Elkin 1994, 160; Meggitt 1962, 389; Mobbs 1991, 316; Tonkinson 1982, 239; Willis 1985, 28).

Some researchers suggest that the lack of biomedical knowledge possessed by many Aboriginal people leads them to credit local healing techniques with which they are more familiar. Taylor (1977, 39) comments, "a new kind of medical system is not automatically accompanied by new knowledge and understanding about disease." Although Warlpiri people are knowledgeable in regard to some diseases, such as diabetes, others can be unfamiliar. Warlpiri people lacked a greater knowledge of biomedical explanations, in part, because medical staff did not always give comprehensive descriptions of illnesses or treatments. During his time in the clinic, neither of the nurses spoke to George or his family at length about what was occurring inside his body. In instances such as this, it is tempting to understand accounts of sorcery as a way of making sense of illness by using concepts that are readily available and understandable. However, this explanation is not completely satisfying. As the previous chapter demonstrated, Warlpiri people are able to use biomedical concepts, such as genetics, without possessing comprehensive biological knowledge. Consequently, it is not necessary to have a firm understanding of biomedical ideas to employ them as explanations or accept their validity.

The tendency of Warlpiri people to credit *ngangkari* after clinical treatment should not be dismissed as simply the result of biomedical ignorance, but rather understood as a meaningful tool through which the value of Aboriginality is articulated. Like diagnoses, claims concerning the efficacy of a specific therapy are capable of expressing notions of race and race relations. As demonstrated earlier in regard to food, the categories of *yapa-kurlangu* and *kardiya-kurlangu* embody the division between Aboriginal and non-Aboriginal histories, people, and traditions. Given that a variety of treatments are often utilized during a single illness episode, it is possible to attribute recovery to a combination of *yapa-kurlangu* and *kardiya-kurlangu* therapies. Yet, in practice, Warlpiri people will credit a single tradition, usually *yapa-kurlangu*. Attributing George's recovery to *ngangkari* is just one example. In the first chapter, James asserted that the *yapa-kurlangu* technique of putting mud on an injury was more effective than attending the clinic, despite having a bandage on his leg. In the second chapter, bush foods were promoted as a cure for diabetes. Similarly, praising the effectiveness of *yapa-kurlangu* techniques affirms the importance and power of Aboriginality. Through health narratives, Warlpiri people negotiate ethnic difference.

Representations and Actions

After his evacuation, George remained at the Katherine Hospital for three weeks, where he received treatment from a variety of medical staff. His condition was carefully monitored and his health began to improve substantially. George was visited by relatives and friends in Katherine, but he missed Lajamanu. When we spoke on the phone, George said that he was feeling much better and wanted to come home. Almost all of Lajamanu's residents disliked hospital stays. While the close care provided ensured that patients physically recovered more quickly than at home, Aboriginal people were socially isolated during this time (Heil 2009). Feeling discomfited, it was not unusual for Warlpiri patients to leave the hospital before they were discharged. While visitors were popular sources of rides back to the community, I knew several people who simply got dressed and walked out the door. Medical staff often referred to this behavior as "absconding," complaining that patients would reappear in the community sicker than when they had left. This would result in another medical evacuation to Katherine. In one instance, a Lajamanu resident left the Katherine hospital three times, only to be returned by plane as soon as the nursing staff spotted him in the community.

Although the social discomfort of hospital stays motivated many of those who departed early, another factor was the lack of treatment for spiritual illness. As George noted prior to attending the clinic, there are no *ngangkari* in hospitals. Patients who do not feel they are getting better or who continue to assert that they are suffering from spiritual disease will attempt to receive treatment from *ngangkari*. As staff generally frown on the use of *ngangkari* in medical facilities, consultations must occur outside the hospital. While it might appear as if assertions of spiritual illness discourage clinical care, this is not necessarily the case. After receiving treatment from *ngangkari*, patients often returned to the hospital of their own volition. Just as George sought a *ngangkari* prior to attending the clinic, others also use *ngangkari* and nurses as complementary options.

When George finally returned to Lajamanu, he had lost about twenty-five kilograms. Speaking positively about the hospital staff that had looked after him in Katherine, he vowed to go to the clinic for monthly checkups to monitor his heart and blood pressure. But as the days passed, George slowly gained back the weight. He predicted that it would not be long before he returned to his former size. After a few weeks, George began to miss appointments at the clinic. Over time, his health began to deteriorate. Suffering from *minta* and other ailments remained a feature of his life. Eventually, Tina's prediction proved to be accurate. Less than two years after this episode occurred, George experienced another severe health crisis and died. In remote Aboriginal communities throughout the Northern Territory, tales such as George's—continual bouts of illness, repeated efforts to obtain treatment, and eventual death—are commonplace.

In recounting George's illness, my goal is not to construct a hierarchy of treatment resort that every Warlpiri person follows, but rather to explore how, during a single illness episode, individuals utilize etiologies and therapies that are commonly referred to as conflicting and discrete. Focusing only on a purely theoretical understanding of etiologies and treatment regimens, one can easily become convinced that two disparate health systems exist in Lajamanu. However, in practice, this is not the case. Examining individual actions and statements, such as George's, demonstrates the complexity of illness experience. Warlpiri health narratives and behaviors are influenced by a number of factors including popular ideas of Aboriginality, gender norms, familiarity, and feelings of physical discomfort and pain. Idealized models might be used to make sense of a disease and to justify behavior, but actual responses to a particular illness are capable of transcending the prescribed treatment of these models. Social dynamics, symptom type, and resource availability are all variables that can change from illness to illness and, as a result, so do actions. In many cases, illness sufferers are more concerned with the social and physiological consequences of treatment rather than strictly adhering to a consistent explanatory logic. In practice, Warlpiri people make use of one system that employs a variety of beliefs, technologies, and treatment options.

Nevertheless, there is an unfortunate tendency to view Indigenous patients "as deciding between alternative medical systems—rather than choosing from among alternative treatments—as if each were an undifferentiated system of treatment practices" (Welsch 1991, 34). While local conceptions of health do influence how illness is conceived and treated, they should not be reified into a single or rigid Aboriginal system that is contrasted with biomedicine. Assertions such as Sutton's (2005; 2009), which cast sorcery beliefs as a barrier to adopting biomedical explanations and treatment regimens, tend to overlook the intricacies of everyday life. Warlpiri beliefs concerning the division of spiritual and physical illnesses do impact how disease is explained and might even act as justification to delay a trip to the clinic, but they do not automatically prohibit the adoption of clinical explanations or treatment. A diagnosis—whether it is sorcery or heart failure—is only one of many factors that motivate treatment choice. Other considerations, such as social norms and illness experience, will probably have a greater influence on therapy decisions. Consequently, resisting biomedical diagnoses for a particular illness does not necessitate a rejection of biomedical treatments for that illness. There is no rigid link between diagnosis, treatment, and adherence to that treatment. Examining Aboriginal responses to renal disease, Devitt and McMasters (1998, 87) accurately observe, "Patients may both subscribe to preternormal causality *and* adhere—to the best of their ability—to medical treatment; also they may not."

But even as residents of Lajamanu mix etiologies and treatments, perceptions of difference continue to structure illness accounts. Statements stressing the incommensurability of Indigenous and non-Indigenous traditions, diagnoses, and techniques will no doubt persist in Lajamanu and within medical contexts generally. As long as ethnic difference remains a ubiquitous feature of life, health narratives will continue to reflect this reality. Through dialogues of conflicting medical systems, notions of Indigeneity are perpetuated and contested. As the next chapter will demonstrate, these dialogues are particularly evident within the confines of the clinic, where white nurses expect Aboriginal patients to comply with their instructions. Medicine is a process through which individuals perform and affirm social roles.

CHAPTER 5
Noncompliance

Pharmaceuticals have increasingly become one of the most effective tools to battle disease. However, for many people living in the developing world, the availability of drugs is limited. Although treatments exist for diseases such as HIV and tuberculosis, their high cost restricts use. The World Health Organization (2004) estimates that over one third of the world's population is denied regular access to medicine. The distribution of pharmaceuticals has become a global health priority in the hope of increasing life expectancy in developing nations. In many settings, access to medication is equated with improved health outcomes. But in Australia's Northern Territory, where health care and prescription drugs are provided free of charge to Aboriginal residents of remote communities, these individuals continue to suffer from the poorest health in the nation. This chapter reevaluates the assumption that access to pharmaceuticals inevitably results in improved health and illustrates the ways in which structural, experiential, and social contexts imbue medication with multiple meanings.

Pharmaceuticals have become a part of everyday life for many people in Lajamanu. Analgesics, cough syrup, and skin ointment were purchased from the shop, while prescriptions were regularly obtained from the clinic. Clinic staff distributed rehydration therapy, skin cream, and antibiotics as well as medication to treat hypertension and diabetes. Given the high rate of chronic illness and morbidity, individuals were often prescribed a variety of pills for extended periods. While pharmaceuticals were widely distributed in Aboriginal communities, nurses complained that a significant percentage of residents were "noncompliant." Compliance has been defined as "the extent to which an individual's behavior—in terms of taking medication, following diets, or executing lifestyle changes—coincides with medical or health advice" (Jay, Litt, and Durant 1984, 124). The notion of compliance has been critiqued for advocating unquestioning patient submission to authoritative medical guidance while ignoring the political and economic contexts in which pharmaceuticals are situated (Humphery 2006; Rouse 2010). Mindful of this appraisal, I seek to invoke noncompliance as a local idiom—a term that is frequently utilized by medical staff and researchers across the Northern Territory—rather than a universal prescription.

In Lajamanu, noncompliance was most often associated with the use—or rather disuse—of pharmaceuticals. On one of my visits to the clinic, Caroline, a nurse, pointed out five shelves filled to capacity with medications awaiting pick up by patients. This represented prescriptions for approximately 125 people, or about 15 percent of the total population. Every four weeks, boxes containing hundreds of uncollected pills were sent back to Katherine where they were destroyed. As in Lajamanu, high rates of pharmaceutical noncompliance are the norm among Aboriginal people living throughout the Northern Territory (Devitt and McMasters 1998; Mathews 1996; Scrimgeour, Rowse, and Lucas 1997; Taylor 1978). Adherence to some therapies has been found to be as low as 5 percent (Kruske, Ruben, and Brewster 1999).

During conversations with medical professionals, excessive rates of noncompliance were blamed for many of the health problems that plagued the Aboriginal population. I was told that noncompliance can allow a disease to worsen, resulting in an increased risk of hospitalization or permanent health damage. Failing to control diabetes can lead to a loss of limbs or eyesight, while not taking a full course of antibiotics has caused the emergence of resistant strains (Mathews 1996, 32). In addition, noncompliance costs health services a great deal. Medical staff expend valuable time and resources treating diabetes complications and other conditions that are considered preventable if pharmaceuticals are taken regularly. The expense of discarding unused pills and funding emergency plane evacuations is one reason that the Northern Territory consistently spends larger per capita sums on Aboriginal health. In an effort to curb the financial and health costs, research has been conducted into the factors that contribute to high rates of noncompliance. In many cases, structural dynamics such as inadequate storage facilities, misunderstandings between nurses and patients, and overwork are blamed (Cramer 2005; Humphery 2006). While there is no doubt that these issues frame responses to medication, the situation is far more complex than most health professionals acknowledge.

The distribution, conceptualization, and utilization of pharmaceuticals are meaningful acts through which relationships—local and international—are constructed and articulated (Farmer 1999; van der Geest and Whyte 1989; Whitmarsh 2008). Pharmaceuticals are not simply objects that are supplied, stored, and consumed. They are inherently social. Examining clinical consultations, van der Geest (2005) asserts that medicines function as a sacrament—a physical instantiation of belief. Prescriptions embody the relationship between the caregiver and care-receiver. Through medicinal interactions our values and convictions are confirmed. By giving cough syrup to a sick child, a mother treats physical symptoms while simultaneously affirming her role as a nurturer (Whyte, van der Geest, and Hardon 2002). Similarly, a rejection of pharmaceuticals in favor of local plant medicines can act as a commentary on globalization (Wayland 2004).

In a setting where non-Indigenous people continue to provide the majority of medical care to an Indigenous population, pharmaceuticals not only establish associations between caregivers and care receivers, they also build upon existing relationships between non-Indigenous and Indigenous people. In Lajamanu, every box of uncollected pills embodies interactions between Aboriginal and non-Aboriginal people. Pills become a physical locus through which social identities surrounding Indigeneity can be performed, negotiated, and resisted. While ostensibly concerned with the disuse of pharmaceuticals, nursing narratives of noncompliance also display and entrench non-Aboriginal attitudes regarding Aboriginality. Warlpiri people, in contrast, never refer to themselves as noncompliant. Instead, their pharmaceutical narratives tend to focus on the attitudes and behaviors of medical staff. These dialogues are shaped by the structural and experiential circumstances of illness and clinical treatment.

"Too Many Pills"

As Caroline pointed out the rows of prescription boxes waiting to be picked up, she stated that noncompliance resulted, in part, from current trends in health service delivery: Possessing little in depth knowledge of the community, non-Aboriginal medical staff routinely prescribed several medications to patients who did not always comprehend their instructions. Caroline's perspective is supported by a great deal of research that demonstrates that misunderstood instructions, frequent changes in staff, and short consultations affect rates of compliance across Australia (Cramer 2005; Damien 1998; Hamrosi, Taylor, and Aslani 2006;

Harrington et al. 2006; Saethre 2005; Saethre 2007b). In an effort to address these issues, medication for Aboriginal people was specially packaged to help ensure that the appropriate dosage was taken at the appropriate time. Each prescription box contained one week of medication. Inside, the pills were sorted into small plastic sachets labeled either "b'fast," "lunch," or "tea." Nursing staff instructed patients to take the entire contents of one sachet at the appropriate meal.

Caroline complained that much of the misunderstandings regarding dosage occurred because of what she termed "over-prescribing." Showing me the contents of a medication box, she pointed to a charcoal pill that was often given to settle digestion. Caroline commented that, in her opinion, this was unnecessary. If people were having digestive problems, remedies purchased from the shop could be used as an alternative. This would allow individuals to self-medicate as needed, while saving the clinic money. But Caroline did not believe that current clinical practices would change. Many of the nurses in Lajamanu blamed doctors for habitually prescribing far too many medications. Physicians based in Katherine— who arrived by plane and stayed for only a couple of days—were considered the worst offenders. These itinerant doctors were characterized as exclusively relying on medical charts rather than trying to understand the personalities and social circumstances of individual patients.

Nursing staff also criticized physicians for having unrealistic expectations regarding rates of pharmaceutical adherence. If given the choice between administering an injection or prescribing medication, many nurses expressed a preference for injections to avoid possible noncompliance. In contrast, doctors tended to favor prescriptions, even when patients expressed a disinclination to take them. After a drug was prescribed, the responsibility of policing compliance often fell to nurses: Brian, a nurse, complained that Kendra, a Katherine-based doctor, instructed him to ensure that a reluctant patient took his medication as directed. Brian replied that this was impossible. Kendra repeated the phrase "make him do it" until Brian walked out of the room in frustration. The following day, Kendra boarded a plane bound for Katherine and did not return for two weeks.

An already difficult situation was further complicated because non-Aboriginal medical personnel rarely served in Lajamanu for extended periods. Physicians and nurses tended to come and go with alarming frequency. Caroline commented that doctors new to the community often ignored previously established regimens and significantly altered existing medications. With frustration, she remarked that a new doctor had just been sent from Katherine and would probably not respect an agreement that the nurses had made with one noncompliant patient. After talking with the patient and an Aboriginal Health Worker, the nursing staff decided to stop ordering medication for him. Caroline noted that each time the man consulted a new physician, a new set of medications were prescribed, which he would not take. Like other medications that are not collected, the patient's latest pills will be discarded and nursing staff could be reprimanded for not ensuring his compliance.

Even patients who attempted to take their medication regularly could encounter confusion over dosage, particularly when antibiotics and analgesics were prescribed together. Caroline remarked that it was difficult to explain that the former must be taken regardless of symptoms, whereas the latter should only be used if the patient was experiencing discomfort. Not only was English a second language for most Warlpiri people, nurses generally spent only a short time with each patient due to the large number of people consulting the clinic on a daily basis. The clinic logbook recorded that over 70 percent of all consultations lasted fifteen minutes or less. Regardless of the steps made to simplify instructions, communication between nurses and patients continued to be a major barrier, especially given the large number of pills that were distributed to each individual.

Despite attempts to curb misunderstandings regarding dosage by providing Aboriginal patients with clearly labeled sachets, this system did not always function successfully. Caroline described a recent experience with a hypertensive patient whose blood pressure had not decreased despite claims of taking medication regularly. After inspecting the patient's prescription box, Caroline discovered that it contained fourteen "b'fast" sachets instead of the usual seven. Other nurses in the clinic were also baffled at the abnormal number. Eventually, Caroline learned that because each sachet could only hold a limited amount of pills, patients who were given numerous prescriptions received multiple sachets for a single meal. Caroline's patient should have been taking two "b'fast" sachets each morning, but only one "lunch" and one "tea" later in the day. Due to the misunderstanding, the patient had not been getting an adequate dose. When informed of the situation, the patient was upset that her health could have been put at risk because of the ignorance of clinic staff. Caroline asked, "How can we expect the patients to comply when even the nurses can't figure it out?"

While medical interactions between Aboriginal people and non-Aboriginal medical staff often take center stage, hierarchies within the clinic and hospital also impact how and why pharmaceuticals are distributed. Although nurses and doctors worked together as part of a medical team, their responses to noncompliance could differ significantly. Their disagreements and misunderstandings had very real consequences on the rate of Aboriginal compliance. Although few Warlpiri people were aware of the complex dynamics that existed between members of the non-Aboriginal medical staff, the preponderance of pills and shifting personnel were often topics of conversation. When asked about her prescriptions, one woman succinctly noted, "There are too many pills." John, like other Warlpiri people, commented that one reason he did not take medication was that it seldom remained the same from month to month, "It is all mixed up." In a community where an egalitarian ethos and social economy drive expectations and actions, seemingly authoritarian instructions given by transient non-Aboriginal workers hold little sway. Despite being given kinship designations, few non-Aboriginal staff participated in Warlpiri sociality or reciprocity. There was little social motivation for Warlpiri people to follow instructions that would change once a new *kardiya* arrived at the clinic. While the nursing staff tended to accuse doctors of failing to establish long term relationships and understandings with Aboriginal patients, from a Warlpiri point of view this was true of almost all non-Aboriginal personnel.

Symptoms

In Lajamanu, medical staff and Warlpiri people used very different criteria to determine if medication was needed. While nurses and doctors often relied on the statements of patients to establish the severity of an illness, in some instances medical tests were performed, such as monitoring the blood sugar of diabetics. These empirical assessments significantly impacted the perceptions of medical staff. When discussing the incidence of chronic illness with nurses or doctors, I was almost always told that the glucose levels of diabetics were exceedingly high. In some cases, I was given quantitative data to support these assertions. One nurse reported that over a two week period, every diabetic she tested had blood sugar concentrations over 18 mmol/1. Given that these levels should be less than 10 mmol/1 following a meal and between 4 to 6 mmol/1 when fasting, it seemed obvious to medical staff that these individuals desperately needed medication. I was told that levels higher than 18 mmol/1 would "debilitate a white person," yet nurses acknowledged that Aboriginal diabetics continued to go about their daily lives as if nothing unusual was occurring. While medical staff viewed chronically elevated blood sugar concentrations as proof that a serious medical crisis was plaguing the community, Warlpiri people had a different perspective.

Despite hearing the results of glucose tests, many Warlpiri people experienced diabetes as an abstract idea rather than as an easily recognized set of aches and pains. Although one of the primary symptoms of high glucose levels—headaches—was a common condition in Lajamanu, people were accustomed to enduring this discomfort. While it is difficult to gauge how many of these cases were the result of improperly controlled blood sugar, headaches were never identified as a symptom of diabetes.[1] Instead, they were simply accepted as a normal part of everyday life. Like Martin, who was discussed in the first chapter, most Warlpiri people asserted that their health was good despite having endured years of chronic disease and acute illnesses episodes. Although nurses invoked medical tests as evidence of illness, Warlpiri residents often doubted the accuracy of these diagnoses if they were unable to identify abnormal symptoms. Like many other diabetic residents of Lajamanu, John experienced difficulty keeping his blood sugar under control. While the nursing staff instructed him to have his glucose levels monitored at the clinic at least once a fortnight, John rarely appeared for his scheduled appointment. When he did attend the clinic for blood tests, John was often surprised at the results. After one visit, John remarked that the nurse had clearly misjudged the severity of his condition: "She said, 'You should be in a coma.' But I don't see why. I feel right." John added that she must be "crazy" to believe his health was so poor. Due to a lack of symptoms other diabetics also doubted clinical diagnoses. Martin said, "They [the clinic staff] said I am really sick, but I don't feel anything." Aside from occasionally feeling tired and lethargic, he had no other indications that his body was not functioning properly.

Because diabetes, hypertension, and several other chronic diseases were not linked to recognizable sensations, pharmaceuticals to treat these conditions were not regularly consumed, despite the instructions of medical staff. On one occasion, George commented that because he did not feel sick, he could not see any benefit to taking long-term medication for hypertension at the rate prescribed by the nursing staff. Many Warlpiri asserted that they saw no need to follow a treatment regimen when they did not appear to be ill. A diabetic said, "Sister says I have to take pills but I am strong. I don't need them." After being given medication for high blood sugar or hypertension, some Aboriginal residents asserted that the nursing staff were either poorly trained or incompetent. John asked why he should take pills when the nurses clearly could not give the right diagnosis.

If the symptoms of illness were seldom identified, the positive effects of complying with medication for chronic illnesses were similarly obscure. For instance, when George was first prescribed medicine for hypertension, he reported taking the pills as directed. However, after a few weeks George stopped, claiming that he had not noticed any improvement in his general health or well-being. Likewise, I often heard John complain that the pills prescribed by the clinic had no effect on his health. Examining the relationship between recognizable symptoms and treatment regimen for leprosy in Papua New Guinea, Lewis (1993, 205) writes, "Any long term treatment puts its own merits in doubt because of the wait and the lack of obvious results." Caroline commented that she had only treated one individual who reported noticing an improvement in his health as a result of taking medication to control diabetes. Subsequently, the patient adhered to his pharmaceutical regime and altered his diet, resulting in his blood sugar level dropping from 12 mmol/1 to 6 mmol/1.[2]

Therapies identified as efficacious through personal experience were far more likely to be followed. A few residents of Lajamanu, such as George, encouraged the use of vitamin supplements. As a result, I occasionally received requests for vitamins, most commonly vitamin C. Some of these individuals were skeptical about taking vitamins, but decided to try a few tablets to discover for themselves if the supplements were effective. In some cases individuals reported vitamins noticeably improving their health. One woman asserted that regularly taking vitamin C caused her boils to disappear quickly and prevented new ones from forming. Consequently, she frequently came to my home asking for vitamin C tablets. Although she confessed to initially believing that vitamins were ineffective, her opinion changed as a result of bodily experience. The vitamins, I was told, "worked," unlike pharmaceuticals to control chronic illness. While taking vitamin C tablets, she did not comply with her diabetes medication.

Although neglected in some contexts, pharmaceuticals were nevertheless employed to relieve a variety of complaints. Scabies, severe diarrhea, and high fevers almost always prompted the use of pharmaceuticals. However, once an individual felt that the illness was improving, treatment was often terminated. This was particularly evident with the use of antibiotics. Although patients initially attempted to comply with the frequency and dosage, as their discomfort lessened, clinical guidelines were less stringently followed. Once symptoms disappeared, individuals often discontinued treatment altogether, despite nursing instructions to complete a full dose. One woman reported discarding her antibiotics once her fever and nasal congestion began to subside, stating that she felt cured and consequently no longer required drugs.

Dangerous Pharmaceuticals and Alternative Treatments

While many Warlpiri people suffering from chronic illnesses were reluctant to consume their medications because they did not recognize the severity of these conditions, individuals were also concerned about possible side effects and other negative consequences associated with the repeated use of pharmaceutical drugs. Parents often worried that their children would accidently swallow adult medications. In Lajamanu, living spaces were often considered communal, locks on doors seldom worked, and secure storage facilities were rare. Consequently, household residents had few effective options for protecting valuables or medications from the hands and mouths of inquisitive children. Brightly colored pills could be mistaken for candies. Nurses recounted stories of children rushed to the clinic after having consumed medications prescribed to their diabetic parent. In an effort to keep her children away from insulin and syringes, one diabetic woman stored her kit on a high shelf. However, every time that she required an injection, she had to climb precariously on a chair and then reach to the back of the shelf. Even those who took such precautions worried that keeping medications at home could endanger the lives of their children.

Even when taking one's own medication, adults expressed concerns about possible side effects and dangers. A distinction was often made between pharmaceuticals taken sporadically, such as analgesics or scabies cream, and those used to treat chronic illness. Although John took paracetamol to relieve aches, pains, and fevers, he explained that the drug would quickly leave his system. In contrast, John described his diabetes medication as "building up." Based on information gleaned from health programs and news reports on television, John asserted that it was a scientific fact that taking prescription medication for an extended period of time could result in irreparable harm. A belief that long-term use of medication could have a detrimental affect on health was an anxiety echoed by Aboriginal people across the Northern Territory (Humphery, Dixon, and Marrawal 1998, 100). Tim affirmed these concerns, stating that diabetes medication makes patients weak, leaving sufferers with more discomfort than they had before beginning treatment. He added that many *kardiya* medicines have this effect. In some cases, even a limited dose of pharmaceuticals could have an adverse result. A *ngangkari* blamed a short course of medication for blocking his kidneys, resulting in the permanent loss of *nguwa*.

As an alternative to pharmaceutical regimens, many individuals vowed to eat bush foods or utilize plant remedies. While a diet of hunted or gathered local foods is considered an effective treatment for illnesses such as diabetes, most bush medicines are used externally and referred to as either "sniffing" or "rubbing" medicines. Sniffing medicines are most often prepared in hot water and inhaled, whereas rubbing medicines are applied to skin abrasions and other dermatological maladies. In Lajamanu, the most commonly used sniffing medicine is *juju minyiminyi* (*Pterocaulon sphacelaturn*), a low bush possessing small pale green leaves that are attached to long stems radiating out of the ground. The leaves give off a strong menthol scent and are used primarily to treat sinus congestion accompanying *minta*. But as with bush foods, individuals rarely gathered or used bush medicines. Among a sample of Lajamanu residents older than fifty, 76 percent reported familiarity with bush medicines but less than 2 percent had taken bush medicines in the two weeks prior to the survey, compared to 56 percent who reported taking prescribed medicines during this period (Sevo 2003, 305). Whereas I occasionally witnessed residents utilizing *juju minyiminyi* to clear congestion, I never observed the use of rubbing medicines. Bush medicines were not used more frequently because they were much more difficult to obtain than pills. There was no place in the community where medicinal plants could be bought and gathering bush medicines was time-consuming and required resources such as a car and petrol. Nevertheless, lack of use did not discourage individuals from praising bush medicines.

Classified as *yapa-kurlangu*, bush medicines are frequently extolled when compared with *kardiya-kurlangu* pharmaceuticals. Warren, a diabetic, commented that while he occasionally took prescription medication to control his blood sugar, he preferred to eat bush foods instead. Like others, John reported preferring to eat bush foods or take bush medicines as an effective form of treatment for most physical diseases. Steve said, "You take all of those pills from the shop and nothing happens but after using bush medicine you get better." Individuals in Lajamanu often remarked that *juju minyiminyi* was more natural and effective than Vick's® VapoRub®. Similarly, collecting sap—a rubbing medicine—from certain tree species was promoted as an alternative to collecting scabies cream from the clinic. Furthermore, bush medicines were considered to be healthier because they did not build up, cause weakness, or have unexpected consequences. George often stated that bush medicines were preferable to pharmaceuticals because they did not cause side effects.

In asserting that bush medicines are safer and more efficacious than pharmaceuticals, medical explanations are employed by Warlpiri people to justify an abandonment of certain aspects of clinical protocols, such as an adherence to medication. Questioning the long-term value of non-Aboriginal interventions, these narratives cast health as a result of adherence to Aboriginality, not a regimen of pharmaceuticals. Like narratives of nutrition, Aboriginal choices and actions are justified by invoking notions of science. In both cases, claims regarding the value of Aboriginality are transformed into the medical realm. Although individuals do not always consume bush foods or bush medicines regularly, this does not deter narratives praising the curative effects of these items. Furthermore, through stories of crazy nurses, toxic pharmaceuticals and efficacious bush medicines, Warlpiri people portray their decisions to disregard medical advice as rational and responsible. I was seldom told that people simply forgot to take their medicine. Instead, many justifications stressed Aboriginal agency, whereby individuals made conscious and informed choices. These explanations differed significantly from those of the nursing staff.

Complaints of Irresponsibility

While the absence of noticeable symptoms and the danger of pharmaceuticals pervaded Warlpiri discussions of compliance, nursing narratives often focused on the attitudes of Aboriginal people. Noncompliance was a popular topic among medical staff in Lajamanu. Although some nurses, such as Caroline, blamed frequent changes of medication and ambiguous instructions, these explanations were far less common than those highlighting the irresponsibility of Warlpiri people. Members of the nursing staff often asserted that Warlpiri health behaviors were the result of a dependence on care provided by non-Aboriginal people. Tina commented, "The biggest problem is that *yapa* do not look after themselves." Across Australia, nurses have portrayed Aboriginal people as passive (Harrington et al. 2006), lacking initiative and self-help (Mobbs 1991, 314), having acquired a "learned helplessness" (Public Accounts Committee 1996, 22), and adopting a "total dependence on nurses" (Cramer 2005, 57). Humphery (2006) notes that during the Rethinking Compliance project in the Northern Territory, non-Aboriginal nursing staff tended to largely ignore factors such as poverty, the continuing effects of colonialism, and the bureaucracy of medical service provision, while making generalized statements of Aboriginality which stressed the inability of Aboriginal people to act in a timely fashion and prioritize health regimens.

Nursing criticisms of Aboriginal behaviors are principally situated around compliance, presentation, and the ensuing ill health that these actions were assumed to precipitate (Cramer 1995, 2005; Cutter 1976; Damien 1998; Taylor 1978, 42). Iris said, "No one cares enough about themselves to do what is right and take their medication. There are diabetics here that are going to lose their sight because they won't take their pills. Aboriginal people need to learn to take responsibility." I was often informed that blindness, amputations, heart attacks, strokes, and kidney failure would all be dramatically reduced and life expectancy would be dramatically increased if only Aboriginal people would comply. Medical staff complained about residents like George who failed to take prescribed pills for chronic illness and subsequently suffered health crises. Tina told me, "I can give you a list of people who will be dead in five years because they don't take their pills. We are supposed to look after them but how can we if they don't want to live?"

While high rates of pharmaceutical noncompliance were often invoked as proof of Aboriginal irresponsibility, other actions deemed to be in violation of medical instructions could also be cited, as when Warlpiri residents presented for treatment after the clinic was closed. Although the nurses disliked opening the clinic after hours, they were required to treat emergencies and critical cases regardless of the time. Each night one nurse was on call and responsible for the many consultations that would occur throughout the evening and early morning. Over a twelve-month period, the clinic logbook averaged approximately 310 after-hours callouts per month, a figure that appears to have remained relatively constant for over a decade. While some late night consultations were precipitated by serious health crises, nurses complained that the majority of after-hours calls were made by patients with conditions that could be treated the following day or by individuals who wanted to collect test results or pharmaceuticals. Being awakened in the early hours of the morning by a patient asking for an analgesic was a common experience for those on duty. Consequently, the nursing staff referred to these and other "trivial" consultations as "Panadol callouts." In a few instances callouts were unrelated to health. Late one night George suggested that I go to the clinic to get alcohol and cotton swabs to clean the video player, as mentioned previously.

When awakened for a "non-lethal" complaint, nurses often reported wanting to "kill" the perpetrator. Tina asked, "Why should I lose sleep when they are just being lazy?" If a callout was deemed inappropriate, the nurse on duty would often refuse treatment, only to complain the following day about the careless health behavior of Aboriginal residents. After being roused the previous evening, Tina remarked, "A baby could have a temperature all day but they just play cards. When it is night that is when they come. They don't care at all." Before emerging from their flats, nursing staff demanded that the symptoms be described to ascertain if care is urgently needed. Some staff stated that Warlpiri people purposely portrayed their symptoms in a manner that prompted the nurse on call to commence an examination. In a few instances, individuals turned away from the clinic for malingering had to be evacuated to the hospital because they were, in fact, suffering a serious health crisis.

In response to Aboriginal behaviors considered to be inappropriate, nurses tended to visibly express their frustration during medical exams. When Danny knocked on the door fifteen minutes after the clinic had closed, Tina asked Melissa, the nurse who was responsible for after-hours consultations that evening, if the door should be unlocked. Melissa shrugged and replied that she didn't have that much filing to do so she didn't mind seeing him. As soon as Tina unlocked the door and Danny entered, Melissa's casual demeanor changed. She sternly informed Danny of clinic hours and asked, "What was so important that you couldn't come in sooner?" When Danny replied that he had been sleeping, Melissa flung her hands up into the air. After taking his temperature and a urine sample, which contained blood, Melissa informed Danny that the results would be back in three days. She stressed that next time he must arrive before the clinic closed. Melissa instructed Danny to take Panadol for the fever until his appointment. Danny said he understood. Melissa opened the door but Danny remained in the clinic. Melissa looked at him saying, "Don't know. Can't help." Danny shrugged and left. When she had locked the door, Tina said, "They just can't take care of themselves responsibly. They never leave us alone." Melissa turned to me and said, "He won't be back. They almost never come back. I don't know why we bother when they don't seem to care at all." As predicted, Danny did not return to the clinic to collect his test results.

Clinic staff consistently asserted that their responses to Warlpiri patients—admonishing them to take their medications regularly and attend the clinic in a timely manner—resulted from a desire to save lives. I was often told that because noncompliance could lead to the spread of resistant strains, health crises, medical evacuations and death, Aboriginal people were needlessly endangering their health. Late night callouts were thought to negatively impact the level of care that the clinic provided. After staying up all night, nurses reported being exhausted and drained the following day. The admonitions of the nursing staff could become severe. At a community meeting Tina threatened to send her dogs to attack anyone that came to the clinic at night with a frivolous request. Generally, nurses believed that reprimanding patients was a reasonable and necessary response to any action deemed unhealthy or dangerous. One nurse commented, "You have to make them understand that this is for their own good." Tina acknowledged that those who had not worked in Aboriginal communities had a tendency to view her opinions and conduct as harsh. But given the conditions of Lajamanu and her directive to close the health gap, Tina felt her actions were appropriate. Nevertheless, reproofs could lead to confrontations in the clinic.

Confrontations

When Lucy entered the clinic scabies sores were clearly present on her arms. Tina asked, "Need some of that rubbing stuff for your skin?" Lucy nodded. Tina continued, "Yeah, it looks pretty bad." Tina motioned Lucy over and had a closer look at her body. Opening the cabinet and pulling out a tube of cream, Tina began to explain the proper application procedure. However, Lucy was becoming agitated. "I want a needle," Lucy demanded. Pointing to the bottle, Tina replied, "No needle. You use this one." Lucy loudly explained that in another community the nurses used a syringe to treat her scabies. She added that an Aboriginal Health Worker in Lajamanu employed the same technique on yet another occasion. Losing patience, Tina shouted, "[The health worker] was wrong! If she gave you a needle then she didn't know what she was doing." Bending close to Lucy, Tina added, "Look at me, Lucy, needles only for big sores; this one from scratching." Lucy began to yell that she wanted a needle. Tina firmly refused, saying if Lucy wouldn't behave then she should leave the clinic. Tina added, "Every time I see you Lucy we fight." Shouting in Warlpiri, Lucy stormed out of the clinic covered in scabies sores without receiving treatment. After Lucy left, Tina explained to the others present that it was her clinic. If people didn't behave, they could suffer.

While many clinical consultations occurred without incident, others, like the one described above, also took place.[3] As a result, Warlpiri people often complained that the nursing staff was aggressive and made unilateral decisions regarding treatment. When I asked Catherine to characterize her experiences with the health care system, she replied by describing the events leading up to a recent operation. During an examination medical staff discovered a lump approximately one centimeter long in her thyroid. After two months Catherine travelled to Katherine for further tests. She was informed that the lump had not increased in size during this time. Nevertheless, the medical staff urged her to have the lump removed. Catherine refused. She said that the medical staff "came up with" a story designed to make her capitulate to the surgery. Catherine remarked, "They said, 'It will grow if you go back to Lajamanu so just get it done now.' They think *yapa* are stupid but I know they are wrong." After further conversations with the doctor, Catherine had the operation. However, she described the procedure as "forced" and stated that she had had no real choice in the matter. Catherine added, "They treat us like we are animals."

Patients charged that, because they were Aboriginal, they were given little control over the procedures that were performed upon them. Although the days of police officers bringing noncompliant patients into the clinic for treatment have ended, Warlpiri people continue to portray themselves as dominated by medical staff. Furthermore, accusations of hostility, inequality, and racism permeated Warlpiri tales of biomedical treatment. For instance, after undergoing a colostomy in an urban hospital, Martin reported that the white man in the neighboring bed seemed to have the same condition but healed much faster. Martin said, "He didn't get a [colostomy] bag like this. He didn't have a big scar. Nothing."

Martin attributed this difference to racism, asserting that white people receive a higher quality of care than do Aboriginal people. Moreover, Martin claimed that medical staff conduct experiments on Aboriginal people and use the knowledge that they gain to benefit white Australians. Statements drawing attention to perceived racial prejudice also pervaded dialogues concerning pharmaceutical treatments: After John reported that the nurses were "cheeky" and "growled at him" for not taking his medication, he added that this behavior was the result of racism.[4]

Whereas nurses responded to what they perceived to be Warlpiri noncompliance by scolding patients, Aboriginal people often reacted by verbally confronting medical staff. Catherine stated that the rampant racism and coercion from medical staff forced her to "speak up." This often entailed cursing at the nursing staff. Many of the residents in Lajamanu described shouting obscenities while obtaining treatment. Nurses were called "cunt" or told to "fuck off." When John returned from the clinic one afternoon, he reported that the nurses had not prepared his insulin injection. Angry, he complained that they expected him to be compliant but did not have his injection ready. John said, "I had to tell her 'fuck you.'" He immediately left the clinic without receiving his blood test or injection. Cursing occurred so frequently in the clinic that Sharon, referring to the kinship system used in many Aboriginal communities, declared, "My skin name is white cunt!"

Nursing staff across the Northern Territory are accustomed to being the target of verbal confrontation as a part of their daily routine (Cramer 1995, 2005; Robins 1996; Scheppers et al. 2006). While nurses and doctors in Lajamanu were most often the recipients of verbal aggression, on rare occasions more severe incidents occurred, ranging from home break-ins where feces were smeared over the walls to attempted assault. In a survey, remote area nurses reported experiencing the following types of violence: verbal aggression (79.5 percent), property damage (31.6 percent), physical violence (28.6 percent), sexual harassment (22.5 percent), stalking (4.9 percent), and sexual abuse/assault (2.6 percent) (Opie et al. 2010, 20). Well aware of the frequency of aggressive encounters, the Territory Health Services ended a two-week cross-cultural training course by discussing violence and teaching self-defense (Lea 2008, 109).

"Cultural violence" perpetrated by nursing staff—such as the transgression of a community norm—is routinely blamed for precipitating Aboriginal violence (Cramer 2005, 66; Robins 1996, 133). While gender norms regulated most day-to-day interactions in Lajamanu, some female members of the non-Aboriginal medical staff chose to ignore these social rules. For instance, many aspects of male reproductive health were considered to be men's business. Warlpiri men asserted that it was shameful and inappropriate to discuss these issues with women. Due to the chronic lack of male medical practitioners in Lajamanu, the only way to see a male doctor or nurse was often through a referral to Katherine hospital. Rather than sending patients into town, female clinicians would occasionally insist on treating men's conditions themselves. In most cases, the doctor or nurse was aware that she was breaking an important gender norm. This behavior could result in severe consequences. When examinations or treatment thought to be gender inappropriate took place, harassment of the medical staff or even attempted assault could occur. Given this example, it appears as if blaming non-Aboriginal cultural violence for Aboriginal physical violence is reasonable. But like other explanations, it attempts to make sense of violence in Aboriginal communities by focusing on the exceptionality and inflexibility of Aboriginal culture. Lea (2008) notes that nurses often assume that violence is confined to remote Aboriginal communities where culture is believed to be strongest. She (Lea 2008, 113) writes, "Terror has to have both a home and a cause—and not just any old causal analysis will do. It must be treatable and even preventable, given the right collaborative diagnosis and sensitive approach." In trying to formulate solutions to high rates of violence against nurses, lessons regarding culturally appropriate behavior reify and perpetuate prevailing conceptions of Aboriginality, while ignoring the larger context of social relations.

Examining confrontations in Bourke, Cowlishaw (2004) characterizes interactions between Aboriginal and non-Aboriginal people as a type of performance which is intentional and enacted in response to an audience. She notes that tension between Aboriginal and non-Aboriginal people is a source of racial identity and motivation. Through complaints of irresponsibility and racism, individuals construct and entrench notions of race. Furthermore, Cowlishaw (2004, 60) observes, "agency is derived from injury." Aboriginal people invoke evidence, such as complaints of white racism, to motivate action, such as cursing at a policeman. Similarly, white shop owners invoke evidence of crime and vandalism to bar the entry of Aboriginal children who are unaccompanied by an adult. Aboriginal people collect and circulate confirmations of white malice, while non-Aboriginal people marshal testimonies of Aboriginal irresponsibility. In these instances, Aboriginality and whiteness are respectively performed. Expanding upon Cowlishaw's notion of agency, her insights are particularly germane to understanding clinical interactions.

Through the process of medical treatment, nursing staff demonstrated ethnic identity. By altering their behavior, vocabulary, and intonation in very specific ways in response to their audience, nurses enacted whiteness. Although medical staff were informed of Warlpiri gender norms through experience, cultural awareness training, or the comments of community members, ignoring these customs publically demonstrated the difference between Aboriginal and non-Aboriginal people. Reflecting on a conversation with an Aboriginal woman in which she was told that her clothing was too revealing, one nurse commented, "They don't do what I tell them, so why should I change for them?" Another added, "This is Australia and I can wear what I like no matter what these people think. It's their community but it's my country."

While nurses chided Warlpiri people and disregarded social rules, they adopted very different mannerisms when speaking to other non-Aboriginal people. An inclusive language that stressed tacit understandings was often employed that used phrases like "you know how they are." These statements mirrored narratives of Aboriginal inaction that occurred regularly among non-Aboriginal workers in Lajamanu. Whether talking to each other in the clinic, relaxing at a non-Aboriginal social gathering, or sitting at home having tea with friends, medical staff repeatedly cast Warlpiri people as unreliable. If I was present when Aboriginal people were obtaining treatment, nursing staff would often complain about the behavior of the patient while explaining the diagnosis to me in detail. Meanwhile, the nurse would tell the Warlpiri patient that he or she had not followed directions, had come at the wrong time, or had in some way not acted as a responsible individual should. Interactions such as these publically reinforced the social differences between non-Aboriginal and Aboriginal people.

When stressing the importance of following biomedical protocols, most of the nursing staff envisioned health being improved through Aboriginal behavioral change—taking pills, increasing nutrition, enhancing hygiene. Aboriginal people, they said, needed to take individual responsibility. Macro-level factors like structural violence and social exclusion were notably absent. Furthermore, despite being largely unproven, the assumption that higher rates of compliance resulted in lower rates of disease was ubiquitous among medical staff. Reflecting a specific type of sociality, biomedical beliefs regarding the importance of compliance have been linked to Western notions of personal responsibility and the authority of medicine (Gordon 1988; Gordon 2000; Reiser 1985; Wikler 1987). At its heart, compliance is a narrative about moral citizens yielding to the expertise and knowledge of medical practitioners. While Aboriginal beliefs and practices are given a great deal of attention and cast as a potential barrier to behavioral change, the assumptions that underlie the compliance narrative are overlooked.

Although racial ideas are expressed in nursing narratives nurses sought to avoid accusations of bias by maintaining that these attitudes are motivated by a commitment to lowering rates of Aboriginal morbidity and mortality. Medical staff, like Tina, often argued that their own aggressive actions were necessary to ensure behavioral change and improve health. Statements invoking medicine, epidemiology, compliance and health disparities often articulated ideas about whiteness and Aboriginality, while claiming to be dissociated from prevailing social stereotypes. Cowlishaw (2004, 35) notes, "while stigma is ascribed to being black, the subtle and symbolic practices that affirm stigma are divorced from blackness." Despite portraying Aboriginal people as irresponsible, the practices that affirmed racial difference—treatment interactions—were recast as unbiased through biomedical discourse. Consequently, narratives of noncompliance are one way in which entrenched, habitual, and constitutive racial rhetoric can be expressed through medical dialogues.

Non-Aboriginal workers were not alone in performing ethnicity. The Lajamanu clinic was a site of active contestation between non-Aboriginal and Aboriginal people. Marshalling evidence of mistreatment at the hands of white medical staff, Warlpiri narratives stressed racial inequality as well as Warlpiri vulnerability to non-Aboriginal control. Portraying their actions as a response to prejudice and domination, Warlpiri people engaged in the performance of Aboriginality through the use of obscenities and other behavior. Conscious of nursing complaints and motivated by assumptions of white racism and Aboriginal disadvantage, Warlpiri people performed popular stereotypes. Constrained by narratives regarding Aboriginal conduct, the forms of expression available to Warlpiri residents were limited. Consequently, Warlpiri people enacted an Aboriginality that was the product of non-Aboriginal discourse. Nevertheless, through an unrelenting repetition of these stereotypes, Aboriginal people were able to contest their meaning. As Butler (1997, 40) notes, "the very terms of resistance and insurgency are spawned in part by the powers they oppose." Behaviors considered by non-Aboriginal people to be inappropriate, such as swearing, become normalized and transformed into an act of defiance.

After confrontations occurred in the clinic, tales of these altercations circulated around the community. Individuals like John and Catherine reported their responses and the reactions of the nursing staff. Stories were often told while discussing the events of the day, with residents supplementing the tales of others with their own. Telling and retelling stories of "speaking up" against presumed injury was an important form of social action. Through medical treatment, the use of pharmaceuticals, and tales of these incidents, Warlpiri people performed Aboriginality and negotiated their identity vis-à-vis non-Aboriginal people.

While most research on issues of Aboriginal adherence to pharmaceuticals has concentrated on biological outcomes such as shortened life expectancy and the creation of resistant viral strains, there is more at stake. In Lajamanu, responses to pharmaceuticals and clinical treatment have become a nexus through which social relationships are executed. Non-Aboriginal nurses and Aboriginal patients enacted ethnicity within the context of everyday life. Attitudes and behaviors surrounding pharmaceuticals and medical advice constituted a forum in which whiteness and Aboriginality were performatively situated within the prevailing social environment. From the perspective of medical staff, the injury of Aboriginal noncompliance was marshaled as evidence for chastising patients. However, these reprimands constituted an injury of their own. Warlpiri people responded, in part, through verbal and physical aggression. In reply, some non-Aboriginal medical personnel cited the intractable behavior of Aboriginal people and ignored Warlpiri social norms. This led to renewed Aboriginal complaints of injury. A seemingly never-ending cycle of injury and agency was perpetuated through the process of medical treatment.

CHAPTER 6
Imposed Empowerment

Despite the existence of comprehensive health care facilities throughout economically developed nations, Indigenous residents continue to suffer from poorer health than non-Indigenous residents. The sporadic and unsuccessful utilization of clinics and hospitals is often attributed to cultural difference and marginality. Because many health services were set up by non-Indigenous governments, are run by non-Indigenous people, and rely on non-Indigenous protocols, it is believed that they are capable of confusing and alienating Indigenous people. To redress the pervasive inequities of treatment, health care initiatives have begun to stress the importance of Indigenous empowerment within a clinical care environment. Empowerment is commonly defined as the process through which individuals, groups, or communities are able to gain increased knowledge and power about decisions and actions affecting their lives. By granting a greater role to Indigenous knowledge, practitioners and ways of life, it is hoped that health care will be utilized more regularly and effectively.

Around the globe Indigenous empowerment through and within health care has become a principal objective. In the United States, medical professionals are urged to address the "cultural barriers to help empower Native American patients" (Oropeza 2002, 1). During his keynote address at the Te Ohu Rata o Aotearoa Māori Medical Practitioners Association Conference, Dr. Mason Durie (2009) urged Māori health leadership to "transform health care into health empowerment." These appeals seek not only improved health outcomes, but also an acknowledgement of social and cultural difference. Empowerment is a strategy for well-being and self-determination that explicitly combines medicine and the politics of Indigeneity. Consequently, understanding the creation, management, and outcomes of these initiatives illustrates the complex relationships between state governments, health professionals, and Indigenous people.

In Australia, widespread dissatisfaction with government health services, living conditions, and economic opportunities has led to repeated calls for Aboriginal empowerment and self-determination. Projects promoting self-determination are often firmly grounded in the belief of cultural exceptionalism, which cast Aboriginal people as fundamentally different (Christen 2009, 8; Cowlishaw 2010, 53). Beginning in the 1970s, increasing attention was focused on improving health through greater Aboriginal involvement in health services. One of the largest results of this effort was the introduction and expansion of the Aboriginal Health Worker Program, which seeks to train and employ Aboriginal people as clinicians working alongside nurses. By the 1980s, notions of self-determination led to the widespread assumption that Aboriginal people would eventually control many aspects of service provision (Christen 2009). In providing Aboriginal people greater input into the delivery of medical care, community controlled clinics have been subsequently indorsed by governments, health care professionals, and Aboriginal people.

Although the Aboriginal Health Worker Program and community controlled clinics seek to increase Aboriginal participation in the health care sector and provide culturally appropriate treatment, they are driven by two different approaches. Modeled after the World Health Organization's village health workers program, the Aboriginal Health Worker Program seeks to combine Aboriginal and non-Aboriginal perspectives. To produce culturally and clinically effective service, the program attempts to promote equality between Aboriginal health professionals and nursing staff. In contrast, community control withdraws participant clinics from government management, allowing them to be run by an Aboriginal board. Community control "braids together calls from Aboriginal advocates for greater autonomy in running Aboriginal health services with a government desire to in fact have less responsibility for (difficult and often futile) arenas of direct service delivery" (Lea 2008, 41). Instead of working in tandem with the governmental health system, Aboriginal people are encouraged to develop their own independent facilities and services.

In Lajamanu, the clinic offers employment to Aboriginal Health Workers and has been community controlled by the Katherine West Health Board since 1998. Despite the goals of equity, empowerment, and better health service provision, the operation of clinic has changed very little. Nurses and patients continued to have disagreements. Many of the stories related in the previous chapter occurred while the clinic was under community control. Aboriginal Health Workers were often dissatisfied with the attitudes and behaviors of non-Aboriginal medical staff and some preferred to be unemployed rather than work at the clinic. Non-Aboriginal medical staff, initially optimistic that Aboriginal control would make a difference, frequently left complaining that Warlpiri people did not show an interest in "taking over" the clinic.

If community control was intended to bring about improvements in medical service delivery within Lajamanu, why did the clinic remain a site of conflict? Furthermore, why aren't more Warlpiri people stepping up to take over the clinic now that it is "theirs"? Examining the Aboriginal Health Worker Program and community control in Lajamanu offers insight into the ways in which notions of Indigeneity are marshaled by the state to govern the lives of Indigenous people. Ultimately, dialogues and initiatives designed to precipitate self-determination had their origins well away from Indigenous communities. Although the goal of community control was to relinquish management to Aboriginal people, in Lajamanu this was achieved through the intervention of the government. Warlpiri people did not respond to these initiatives as many had hoped, partly because this notion of empowerment was not necessarily their own. Warlpiri political processes stress the autonomy of the individual rather than submission to a hierarchy. Consequently, a seeming disinterest in the management of the clinic was, in fact, a powerful expression of Indigenous agency.

The Aboriginal Health Worker Program and "Two Way" Medicine

The roots of the Aboriginal Health Worker Program are embedded in the history of colonialism and its aftermath. Initially, missionaries and governments supplied colonial health services and personnel, but as Europe began to divest itself of its colonial possessions after the Second World War, newly independent African and Asian nations were faced with a shortage of clinical health providers. In these regions, trained health professionals were rare and often reluctant to practice in rural areas. In an effort to provide adequate health care without the long hours of training required to be a nurse or doctor, the World Health Organization began village health worker programs. Basic clinical training was given to local residents in nations such as India, Tanzania, Niger, and Papua New Guinea (Devanesen 1982, 14).

Throughout the various national incarnations of these programs, two distinct types of health workers were created: a medical auxiliary and a primary health care worker (Willis 1985, 40). The former service category was pursued by those intending to achieve a professional clinical award. The candidates were required to have some education, were trained in clinical practice, and expected to work as a nurse's assistant. In contrast, primary health care workers acted as cultural liaisons. Traditional healers were sometimes employed in these positions in hopes of encouraging village residents to utilize the professional health system more frequently and effectively. In almost every instance primary health care workers were selected based upon local community endorsement rather than literacy skills (Willis 1985, 15).

Australian medical personnel working abroad had close and sustained contact with village health worker programs in Papua New Guinea. As nurses returned to Australia, support grew for similar formal training initiatives in the Northern Territory (Kettle 1991, 293). Health services in Aboriginal settlements were continually short-staffed, and nurses saw village training initiatives as a way to supplement medical care in the bush. However, many doubted that Aboriginal people could successfully complete any program that required a comprehensive education. Although missionaries and other service providers regularly instructed Aboriginal people as assistants, this training was informal and focused only on simple diagnosis and treatment techniques (Tregenza and Abbot 1995, 3). Consequently, medical personnel felt that the primary contribution of Aboriginal people would have to be cultural, not clinical. As a result the Aboriginal Health Worker Program was modeled after that of primary health care workers, not medical auxiliaries (Devanesen 1982, 14; Willis 1985, 13). Today medical staff continue to assume that the primary role of Aboriginal Health Workers is that of cultural liaisons (Heil 2006, 105).

The first official health instruction for Aboriginal workers occurred in the early 1950s at East Arm Leprosarium in Darwin, where Aboriginal staff were taught to diagnose and treat Hansen's disease in a three-month course (Josif and Elderton 1992, 11). Although the Leprosarium training was hailed as successful by medical personnel participating in the program, existing laws prohibited Aboriginal people from performing clinical tasks in hospitals, effectively halting further schemes.[1] In addition, there was debate over the venue for formal instruction. Hospitals opposed a proposal to offer clinical courses for Aboriginal people in 1956 and 1958, despite support from the Welfare Branch. It was not until 1959 that the Central Training Establishment was opened in Darwin. A small facility that taught ten to twelve people at a time, it paved the way for subsequent programs (Kettle 1991, 293). By 1965, a Hospital Assistant Course for Aborigines was started at Darwin hospital and in March 1970 the formal requirements for nursing assistants changed, creating the possibility for Aboriginal Health Workers (Josif and Elderton 1992, 11).

In 1973, the first Aboriginal Health Worker course started in Darwin and four years later a similar course began in Alice Springs. Although a course was developed to teach Aboriginal healers clinical practices, it became apparent that it would be better to train a separate group as Aboriginal Health Workers, leaving healers to continue to fulfill their customary roles (Devanesen and Maher 2003, 183). In 1976, Dr. Dayalan Devanesen became the first Coordinator of the Aboriginal Health Worker Training Program in Central Australia. By 1982, a centralized six-week basic skills course was established at the Katherine Institute of Aboriginal Health. It attempted to balance the wishes of non-Aboriginal administrators who favored hospital-based training and Aboriginal students who favored community-based training (Josif and Elderton 1992, 11). Primary clinical instruction would occur in Katherine but it would be supplemented by experience at the student's local clinic. This method ensured that basic standards could be met while also allowing Aboriginal people to gain experience in their own communities, where they preferred to reside. The Aboriginal Health Worker Program was viewed by many as an important victory for Aboriginal residents of the Northern Territory. Aboriginal staff could now provide treatment to their kin in the clinic, whereas previously they were only allowed to sweep the floor (Devanesen 1982, 18).

The Aboriginal Health Worker Program was emblematic of a dramatic change that was occurring throughout the Northern Territory. In the 1970s and early 1980s, there was rising awareness of the need to encourage Aboriginal involvement in the health care system and an acknowledgement of Aboriginal beliefs regarding health and illness. While healers were no longer taught to work in biomedical settings, their expertise was nonetheless acknowledged. In its first policy on Aboriginal health care, the Northern Territory Department of Health states, "traditional medicine is a complementary and vital part of Aboriginal health care, and its value is recognised and supported" (Northern Territory Department of Health 1982 cited in Devanesen and Maher 2003, 183). In an effort to encourage parity and demonstrate the contributions of Aboriginal and Western techniques among clinic staff, Aboriginal Health Workers explained bush medicines to nurses, while nursing staff made a rubbing ointment from wax, fat, menthol, and eucalyptus oil (Devanesen 1982, 20).

By encapsulating these themes, the philosophy of "two way" or "both ways" medicine sought to combine what were believed to be distinct Aboriginal and non-Aboriginal traditions and technologies. Gaining popularity by the late 1970s, the two way philosophy was meant to build bridges within the Northern Territory, allowing for a greater equality and acceptance of Aboriginal practices and lifestyles. While Aboriginal health beliefs had long been acknowledged as an important influence on treatment behavior, two way medicine sought to integrate Aboriginal and biomedical health approaches by incorporating local health customs and practices into clinical protocols. It aimed to promote "traditional healing, hand-in-hand with western medicine" (Northern Territory Aboriginal Health Worker Conference 1988, 6). Under this model, illness management continued to occur in the clinic, although patients could choose to consult nurses or Aboriginal Health Workers, while treatment options would include pharmaceuticals and bush medicines (DaCosta 1996; Grootjans and Spiers 1996). Nursing staff remained primarily responsible for contributing clinical expertise but Aboriginal Health Workers provided cultural knowledge and information to assist in treatment and recovery (Soong 1981, 185). Devanesen (1985, 36) claims that two way medicine bridges "the cultural chasm separating the traditional and western world views."

Two way medicine, coupled with the Aboriginal Health Worker Program, sought to encourage culturally appropriate health care by supporting Aboriginal participation in a medical system that utilized both biomedical and Aboriginal models. With the incorporation of local techniques into formal procedures, Aboriginal residents were to gain an equal voice in health care and a feeling of self-worth. Seeing local traditions like *ngangkari* and bush medicines recognized as effective and valid through their use in the clinic was thought to precipitate community pride in Aboriginal customs and beliefs. The two way movement attempted to improve the self-esteem of Aboriginal people as well as the tolerance of non-Aboriginal health professionals. Furthermore, it was hoped that, as doctors and nurses became accustomed to these practices, a greater acceptance of Aboriginal treatment techniques would result.

One of the main purposes of two way medicine and the Aboriginal Health Worker Program was to improve health outcomes through increased rates of compliance (Josif and Elderton 1992, 11). As with primary health care worker programs in other parts of the world, culturally appropriate care was seen as an important step in encouraging greater use of clinical care facilities. It was hoped that, if clients had kin or someone known and trusted working in the local health center, this would lead to a greater confidence in clinical care, alleviate fears of biomedical treatment, and boost rates of presentation (Willis 1985, 31). Ideally, it was suggested that Aboriginal Health Workers from all major family groups should eventually hold positions in the local health center (Devanesen 1982, 21). In an effort to ensure that respected individuals gained positions in the clinic, community nomination rather than literacy and numeracy skills was initially the primary selection criterion for candidates in the Aboriginal Health Worker Program.

Throughout the 1970s and early 1980s, Aboriginal Health Worker training stressed cultural rather than educational contributions. In the early 1980s, Willis (1985, 16) reports one out of every three Aboriginal Health Workers in the southern region of the Northern Territory was illiterate. Focusing on a list of basic skills, the emphasis was placed on identifying and treating common complaints rather than being able to record large amounts of patient data.[2] One nurse explained the training priorities by noting that, when taking a pulse, Aboriginal Health Workers were taught to feel for any abnormalities, not count how many beats per minute. However, many Aboriginal Health Workers felt that their contributions were valued less than those of doctors and nurses. Cultural skills did not seem to be as highly regarded as clinical ones.

In 1982, the Northern Territory model for Aboriginal Health Workers was recommended as the template for states across the nation (Devanesen 1982, 15). Two years later, the Northern Territory had the highest number of Aboriginal Health Workers in the country and had assigned these individuals a more developed role than in other regions (Thomson 1984, 944). Amidst calls for greater equity with other health professionals, the Northern Territory Health Practitioners and Allied Professionals

Registration Act (1985) certified the Aboriginal Health Worker as an independent professional group. The Northern Territory was the first jurisdiction to have an Aboriginal Health Worker career structure and a professional regulatory board (Northern Territory Department of Health 1998c, 61). In 2004, Aboriginal Health Workers—as well as nurses, midwives, optometrists, and other medical professionals—were regulated under the Health Practitioners Act. In the Northern Territory, Aboriginal Health Workers are required to demonstrate clinical competence in select areas and register with the Aboriginal Health Workers Board. In 2008, the Council of Australian Governments signed an Intergovernment Agreement to create a single national registration and accreditation system for health professionals but Aboriginal Health Workers were left out of the proposal, signaling their unique status.

An important feature of increasing professionalization was an accredited educational facility designed to meet the needs of Aboriginal students. Intended to provide training similar to that of non-Aboriginal institutions, the School of Health Studies at Batchelor College was established in 1990 (Batchelor College 1995). Students completed courses toward their degree at Batchelor, while also gaining experience in their community clinic. In line with the two way philosophy, the method of Aboriginal Health Worker training relied on the successful combination of Aboriginal beliefs and non-Aboriginal techniques, to "Aboriginalise" course content (Josif and Elderton 1992, 12). Now renamed the Batchelor Institute of Indigenous Tertiary Education, the two way philosophy continues to underpin Aboriginal Health Worker training. Students must complete a series of four Primary Health Care certificates before they are eligible to register and seek employment. While the training of Aboriginal Health Workers has been expanded to include specialist areas such as renal dialysis, women's and men's health screening, early childhood screening, nutrition, and mental health, cultural brokerage continues to remain a key responsibility. As Aboriginal Health Workers are being taught to use complex medical equipment and administer drugs, their role as a health care facilitator has not changed.

In moving toward greater professionalization, the Aboriginal Health Worker training regimen has received criticism. For some, formal education in urban centers represents an abandonment of the cultural values that Aboriginal Health Workers are intended to possess in the first place. Saggers and Gray (1991, 163) ask if accreditation is appropriate at all.

They believe that formal education, registered career structures, and standards that may be employed in other skilled sectors could be detrimental to Aboriginal health professionals. It is reasoned that if the primary function of an Aboriginal Health Worker is cultural, then they do not need extensive clinical training. Such a view hinges on a belief that Aboriginal and non-Aboriginal knowledge and technologies are so dissimilar that learning one somehow undermines or destroys the other. These same themes are also present in debates surrounding the presence of *ngangkari* in clinics or hospitals. Opponents charge that Aboriginal healers discourage clinical treatment and should not be incorporated into biomedical care settings (Sutton 2009). As demonstrated in Chapter 4, consulting *ngangkari* does not preclude following clinical regimens. Debates over the presence of *ngangkari* in clinics or the skills training required for Aboriginal Health Workers reflect popular ideas regarding the nature of Aboriginality. To illustrate how these issues have impacted the practical implementation and outcomes of the programs, I turn to the experiences of Aboriginal Health Workers in Lajamanu.

Aboriginal Health Workers in Lajamanu

When I first arrived in Lajamanu, four Aboriginal Health Workers were working at the clinic. Within a few months, they had all resigned. I quickly learned that it was difficult to recruit Aboriginal Health Workers and, even for those already on the job, turnover is high (Department of Health/Department of Aboriginal Affairs, Joint Ministerial Evaluation Team 1982, 252; Josif and Elderton 1992, 48).[3] Although several positions were open and qualified Aboriginal Health Workers continued to reside in Lajamanu, Aboriginal people did not choose to consistently sell their labor. Sometimes employed, sometimes not, the number of Aboriginal Health Workers working in the clinic was seldom constant. On a recent visit, I spoke with an Aboriginal Health Worker staffing the clinic. She said, "I am the only one now."

Across the Northern Territory, Aboriginal Health Workers sporadically begin, resign, and return to employment, with some taking hiatuses of up to ten years (Josif and Elderton 1992, 20; Torr 1988, 29; Tregenza and Abbot 1995, 16). Although approximately 450 Aboriginal Health Workers were registered in 2000, only 195 were employed (Curtin Indigenous Research Centre 2000, 102). In addition to low job retention, the overall number of Aboriginal Health Workers is shrinking. By 2010, the number of registered Aboriginal Health Workers decreased to around 300 (Health Professions Licensing Authority 2010). In an effort to make sense of why this decline has occurred, it is necessary to examine a few of the factors that underlie the experiences of Aboriginal Health Workers, including difficulty completing the educational requirements, conflicts with non-Aboriginal medical staff, and the divergence between medical and community expectations.

For many Aboriginal people in the Northern Territory, the literacy skills needed to become an Aboriginal Health Worker are hard to achieve without remedial classes. Consequently, the level of education necessary to enter the program discouraged some from applying. In one instance, a young man was interested in becoming an Aboriginal Health Worker but was discouraged by the long and difficult application process. Despite these hurdles, he applied for admission, only to give up after failing to receive a timely response from Batchelor. I was told that few people in the community were interested in becoming health workers because completing the requirements was too complex, time consuming, and often required knowledge that they did not possess. The outcomes of a professional and accredited education program requiring literacy and numeracy skills are outweighed, some argued, by its drawbacks.

Despite achieving professional qualifications through education and registration, Aboriginal Health Workers in many community health centers throughout the Northern Territory complained that they were not respected as clinicians, while nurses tended to ignore or see as irrelevant the cultural contributions Aboriginal Health Workers make to the clinic (Damien 1998; Josif and Elderton 1992; Tregenza and Abbot 1995). In Lajamanu, Aboriginal Health Workers often commented that other health care professionals did not respect or trust their abilities. One health worker complained that, after she had examined a baby suffering from a high fever, a nurse asked to review the data she collected, including the baby's weight, temperature, symptoms, and sleeping habits. She felt that the nurse did not treat her as a peer, adding that this made her want to resign from the clinic because she was not valued. Feeling underappreciated was a common sentiment among Aboriginal Health Workers in Lajamanu. Many noted that they were given little input into most issues of service delivery and policy. One said, "We need to talk together, not just get orders." Another agreed and commented that the biggest problem faced by Aboriginal Health Workers was the superior attitude of non-Aboriginal health professionals who did not listen to the advice of community members.

Nursing staff regularly criticized the training, support, and utilization of Aboriginal Health Workers. Because clinical tasks took priority in the health center, nurses and doctors considered the medical knowledge many Aboriginal Health Workers possessed to be limited. Melissa expressed frustration at older Aboriginal Health Workers in Lajamanu because they did not have adequate training and yet, she said, they did not realize this. Melissa felt Aboriginal Health Workers should be required to undergo additional courses at Batchelor where their skills could be updated. Caroline stated that an older Aboriginal Health Worker had not been "trained properly" and needed supervision for most tasks. Nurses across the Northern Territory reported that Aboriginal Health Workers failed to live up to their expectations (Tregenza and Abbot 1995, 28), did not take individual or clinical responsibility (Public Accounts Committee 1996, 150), and were thought to lack initiative and be unsupportive (Taylor 1997, 17). Consequently, some Aboriginal Health Workers were treated as little more than untrained assistants.

The Aboriginal Health Worker Program sought to achieve equity between Aboriginal and non-Aboriginal professionals, but doctors and nurses do not always regard Aboriginal Health Workers as valuable health care professionals. The two way approach that guided the Aboriginal Health Worker Program overlooked the fact that the cultural contributions of Aboriginal Health Workers are not as highly valued in the medical community as formal training. As Curtin Indigenous Research Centre (2000, 16) notes, "There is a basic conflict between retaining a community-involved primary model of health and attempting to attain status and recognition within a medically dominated health service." Consequently, Aboriginal Health Workers often find it difficult to negotiate their own positions and responsibilities (Heil 2006, 105). Instead of being respected for the cultural knowledge they may bring to the workplace, evidence has shown that, without adequate clinical qualifications, Aboriginal Health Workers are often viewed by medical staff as tokens, not equals.

Drawing on popular narratives of Aboriginality in Lajamanu, nurses often portrayed Aboriginal Health Workers as irresponsible. These complaints commonly revolved around absenteeism and use of the clinic's vehicles. I was told of several days when Warlpiri staff did not appear for work. Some of these absences were due to kin obligations. For instance, Aboriginal Health Workers would regularly travel to neighboring communities for funerals and other ceremonies, leaving the clinic short-staffed. In many instances, nurses only learned about these trips at the last minute, if at all. Furthermore, Aboriginal Health Workers rarely returned to work in what the nurses considered to be a timely manner. One nurse joked that the solution to absenteeism was to schedule twice as many Aboriginal Health Workers as were needed to guarantee that enough turned up to provide an adequate level of care.

Another primary point of contention between Aboriginal Health Workers and nursing staff was the utilization of the vehicles used to transfer patients to or from the clinic or airstrip. On occasion Aboriginal Health Workers would either "borrow" the vehicles or "abscond" with them, depending on whether an Aboriginal Health Worker or nurse was relating the story.[4] Nurses complained that one Aboriginal Health Worker often borrowed the clinic van in the middle of the day to do personal shopping or drive kin around the community. I was told that another was notorious for working for an hour or so in the morning and then taking the four-wheel-drive out on personal hunting and gathering trips for the rest of the day, leaving the clinic short-staffed. The health worker claimed that these trips were to collect bush foods—and therefore medicine—for the elderly and expressed frustration over the distrust of the nursing staff.

At times health workers are torn between the expectations of community members and their non-Aboriginal co-workers. While on paper the two primary tasks of Aboriginal Health Workers—cultural awareness and clinical treatment—seem to mesh easily, in actual situations this is not always the case. An Aboriginal Health Worker described an incident that occurred when a senior Warlpiri male entered the clinic expecting to be treated immediately due to his social standing. Conscious that the nurses would be upset if he was treated before the female patients who were already waiting, the Aboriginal Health Worker on duty did not acquiesce to his demand and the man angrily stormed away. After the incident, the man would not allow either a member of the nursing staff or an Aboriginal Health Worker to examine him. His illness worsened as the days passed. Eventually, desperate for relief from severe symptoms, he presented late at night and was evacuated to Katherine Hospital. After the incident, the Aboriginal Health Worker reported being blamed by some community residents for causing the man's illness to worsen. The gender rules, kinship ties, and personal relationships that structure interactions between Warlpiri people in and around the clinic were a potential source of friction. While having family members acting as Aboriginal Health Workers encouraged some to attend the clinic more frequently, this could lead to resentment and allegations from other patients if they felt that preferential treatment was being given. When hostile or customary avoidance relationships existed between an individual and an Aboriginal Health Worker, the clinic could be avoided and utilized only as a last resort. Well aware of these challenges, the Aboriginal Health Worker code of ethics states that Aboriginal Health Workers have a duty to treat all individuals "even in an avoidance relationship" (Health Professions Licensing Authority 2008, 1). Yet when social norms are ignored—for instance, if a senior male is not treated before others in the queue—Aboriginal Health Workers become the target of blame and accusations. These conflicts can have serious consequences for community relationships. Because both patients and Aboriginal Health Workers reside permanently in the community, arguments that begin in the clinic can eventually involve extended family members.

Combining Aboriginal and non-Aboriginal expectations was not as simple as two way medicine promised. In cases where biomedical and Aboriginal protocols seemed to diverge, it was often the former that was followed: treatment was to occur regardless of avoidance relationships. Consequently, Aboriginal Health Workers felt that, in practice, they were clinicians first and cultural brokers second. They provided an extra pair of hands to complete clinical and administrative tasks rather than cultural assistance. Despite assertions that Aboriginal Health Workers and nurses would perform different roles, in reality both provided clinical treatment. Originally intended to handle tasks nurses could not, many Aboriginal Health Workers have become nursing assistants. Their unique role in the clinic has not been realized.

If the concept of cultural liaison is considered it is no surprise that clinical imperatives appear to take priority. What exactly are cultural tasks? Examining the history of the program reveals that Aboriginal Health Workers were originally intended to motivate greater presentation and make the clinical experience more comfortable. It was through the process of treatment itself that local norms were to be supported and affirmed. The cultural aspect of care was demonstrated by the presence of Aboriginal Health Workers and their ability to explain local custom if needed, not in a unique set of protocols or duties. In many instances, "cultural" is simply a gloss for all medical activities not deemed to be "clinical." In this respect, terms such as cultural and clinical—and responses to them—mirror popular notions of Aboriginal and white.

Although the division of the cultural from the clinical has been stressed in the pursuit of parity, the experience of working in the clinic has led Aboriginal Health Workers to share a great deal of common ground with non-Aboriginal medical staff, particularly nurses. Aboriginal Health Workers in Lajamanu often complained that Warlpiri people were too dependent upon the clinic and its services. Echoing statements made by nursing staff, an Aboriginal Health Worker asserted that Warlpiri people were "still there in the welfare days," adding that too often people came to the clinic for minor injuries. The high rate of unnecessary after-hours callouts was also a constant source of grievance. A frequently repeated phrase was "too much humbug." Another health worker stated that the primary obstacle to improved health was a lack of compliance, commenting that too often people wanted to "do things their own way" instead of following the advice of medical staff. Like the nurses, Aboriginal Health Workers asserted that high rates of noncompliance and late presentation were indicative of the irresponsible health behavior of many Warlpiri people. Regardless of these shared views, Aboriginal Health Workers have not been fully integrated into the clinic. Assumptions regarding the division between culture and medicine—as well as arguments over vehicle use and working hours—keep Aboriginal and non-Aboriginal medical staff separated.

Community Control

Although two way medicine and the Aboriginal Health Worker Program were intended to encourage parity, ongoing debates continue over whether this objective was successfully met. In 1997, I spoke with the clinic staff about the effectiveness of two way medicine. Sharon, a nurse with extensive experience working in Aboriginal community clinics, remarked that two way medicine had "never worked" and expressed relief that the Northern Territory seemed to be moving away from this philosophy. In addition to nursing staff, health researchers were increasingly finding fault with two way medicine and its outcomes. Critics charged that the goal of creating a medical environment in which Aboriginal and non-Aboriginal health care traditions coexisted has not been met. Although endorsing a two way model in theory, Burnett (1996, 5) comments that so far only one way has occurred. Nathan and Leichleitner (1983, 68) echo this view, stating the model never operated as described—linking Aboriginal and non-Aboriginal ideals equally. Others state that a merging of systems has yet to truly happen (Humphery, Dixon, and Marrawal 1998, 100).

Researchers, Aboriginal people, and health professionals sometimes cast two way as nothing more than a method of enabling the clinic to enforce the colonial domination of Aboriginal people. According to these views, empowerment through programs such as two way is not about restoring power to Aboriginal people but merely a gloss for conforming to non-Aboriginal standards (Flick 1997, 19). For instance, Saggers and Gray (1991, 150) claim two way medicine is at best a form of tokenism and at worst a tool used by colonizers to appropriate Aboriginal health techniques in an effort to further extend their own non-Aboriginal health care system. They believe that any form of health care that relies on biomedical models, locations, and administrations will not end the domination by the non-Aboriginal health system, no matter how much it incorporates Aboriginal ideals.

Although two way medicine was no longer endorsed with the same intensity, achieving improved medical care through a more equitable medical system remained a priority in the Northern Territory. To meet this goal, a new initiative—local Aboriginal community control of health care facilities—was advocated. Brian felt that community control offered the greatest hope for culturally appropriate service. Whereas two way medicine stressed the importance of Aboriginal participation as clinicians within the larger government health care structure, community control would theoretically allow Aboriginal people to opt out of government service provision entirely. Rather than working as cultural liaisons at the clinic, Aboriginal people would assume management of the facilities. Responsible for making decisions regarding staffing and service provision, the community would have the power to dismiss nurses and offer culturally appropriate treatments. As with other initiatives, the Northern Territory government hoped that community control would increase presentation and compliance rates, thus leading to improved health outcomes (Northern Territory Department of Health 1996, 9).

While community control was relatively new in the Northern Territory, the Aboriginal takeover of health care facilities had successfully occurred elsewhere in Australia. In 1971, the first Aboriginal controlled health service began in Redfern (Thomson 1984, 944). Although there was initial government resistance, this was gradually overcome and the number of community run clinics increased (Katherine West Health

Board 2003, 34). By 1989, the National Aboriginal Health Strategy endorsed community control. The hope was that local health center management would ensure better education and employment opportunities; provide appropriate treatment, cultural support and training for Aboriginal people; and prevent unethical behavior and racism (National Aboriginal Health Strategy Working Party 1989, xvii). A 1996 report on health care provision to Aboriginal people strongly supported the introduction of self-sufficient medical services as a tool for "empowerment/local Aboriginal control" (Public Accounts Committee 1996, 8). That same year, over sixty Aboriginal health services were operating across Australia (Northern Territory Department of Health 1996, 147). These numbers have increased dramatically since that time. Between 1997 and 1998 Aboriginal controlled health services provided an estimated 860,000 episodes of care, but by 2004 this number was over 1.6 million (Australian Medical Association 2002, 6; National Aboriginal Community Controlled Health Organisation 2007, 4).

Historically, the Northern Territory had been home to only a handful of these organizations, most located in urban areas. By the mid 1990s, the Katherine region possessed only three incorporated Aboriginal health services and one community council controlled health service. The Northern Territory government managed the remaining twenty-one rural services, including Lajamanu (Northern Territory Department of Health 1998b, 39). Consequently, many researchers charged that the Northern Territory government was not fulfilling its commitment to encourage and fund locally run medical facilities, regardless of the promises made in health policy statements (Anderson 1996, 16; Bartlett and Legge 1994, 18; Collins and Warcon 1994, 8; Bartlett 1996, 210; Flick and Nelson 1994, 6; Josif and Elderton 1992, 15). Criticized for the pace at which community control was realized, a process to develop these programs was put in place. In 1996, the Commonwealth and Northern Territory governments began negotiations to introduce a comprehensive system of community control and care coordination in some rural regions (Public Accounts Committee 1996, 146; Katherine West Health Board 2003, 36). In addition to sites in the Tiwi Islands (Northern Territory), Wilcannia (New South Wales), and Bunbury/Perth (Western Australia), the Katherine West region was selected to participate in a national scheme of Aboriginal coordinated care trials.

Under the agreement the Katherine West Coordinated Care Trial (KWCCT) would lease the government managed clinics in the region:

Lajamanu, Kalkarindji, Yarralin, Pigeon Hole, Bulla, Mialuni, and Timber Creek. Although coordinated care—the sharing of patient health information between different sectors of health care providers to provide an improved service—had been initiated elsewhere in Australia, this was the first time that Aboriginal communities participated in such a program. These trials were further distinguished because they were specifically designed to provide community control. By involving "Aboriginal people in determining their own health service needs," the effectiveness of primary health care in the region was to be improved (Northern Territory Department of Health 1998b, 31). Community control was realized by transferring clinic management from the government-run Territory Health Services (THS) to the Katherine West Health Board Aboriginal Corporation (KWHB). Comprised of Aboriginal representatives, membership was open to any permanent resident of the trial communities. Shortly after its start, the trial was renamed *Jirntangku miyrta* "One shield for all," to reinforce its "Indigenous identity" (d'Abbs et al. 2000, 16). The trial was launched on 1 July 1998 and was extended until the end of March 2000. After cessation of the trial, the Katherine West Health Board continued to manage the community clinics, making local control a lasting reality.

With the Northern Territory government no longer in control, the KWHB became responsible for appointing service providers, allocating funds, and managing local health centers. This allowed trial communities to obtain renal care, emergency care, and preventative medicine from a variety of providers without having to get clearance from various levels of government (Northern Territory Government 1997, 15). In theory, this would bestow the financial leverage necessary to end inappropriate behavior in local clinics by dismissing nursing staff who failed to respect local norms. The Aboriginal health board would have the ability to employ only health care providers it felt were the most culturally and medically appropriate. An important goal for the health board was redressing the gender imbalance that existed in many clinics (d'Abbs et al. 2000, 82; Katherine West Health Board 2003, 51). It was hoped that better service provision would encourage greater presentation, use of pharmaceuticals, and general health. In addition to increasing Aboriginal participation and health outcomes, the trial was also intended to "empower" Aboriginal community residents (d'Abbs 1998, 17).

The Aboriginal coordinated care trials have been described as "the largest and most ambitious experiment of a new method of organizing healthcare services ever attempted in Australia" (Esterman and Ben-Tovim 2002, 469). The goals of community control and the Katherine West trial were impressive—improved health outcomes and Aboriginal empowerment. While the Katherine West Health Board (2003) reports a decrease in emergency evacuations, an increase in the volume of health services provided, and better rates of staff retention, other evaluations are less positive. Esterman and Ben-Tovim (2002, 469) report, "Despite this effort and expenditure, the outcomes were disappointing. In general, the trials did not demonstrate improved health and well-being of the partici-pants." Though trial evaluators note that Aboriginal people were in con-trol of the health services for the first time, they concede that expectations of client empowerment as a result of the trial was "naïve" (d'Abbs et al. 2000, 85). Lastly, despite a restructuring of health care service provision, the day-to-day challenges facing the Lajamanu clinic were not drastically altered. The final sections of this chapter examine the implementation of Katherine West Trial in Lajamanu to understand why community control did not function as envisioned.

Katherine West

Beginning with my fieldwork in 1996, I witnessed the clinic's transition from a government institution to one that was community controlled. While visiting Lajamanu in 2009 over a decade after the introduction of Aboriginal control, I was struck by how little had changed. Even though the KWHB was managing the clinic, Aboriginal complaints about the medical staff were common, nurses noted that rates of late presentation and noncompliance had not diminished, Aboriginal Health Workers gen-erally chose to remain unemployed, and Warlpiri people stated that they had little or no control in the services that were offered. In examining two central goals of Katherine West—contracting additional health services and providing culturally appropriate treatment—I argue that community control was constrained by an absence of care providers in Australia's rural regions as well as by pervasive assumptions regarding Aboriginal "culture." The policy of local empowerment essentialized ethnic categories, under-estimated the omnipresence of government in Australia's rural regions, and overestimated the interest of Aboriginal people in assuming manage-ment of health care services. Consequently, the material and social circum-stances of rural Aboriginal communities determined outcomes more than did the management by government or an Aboriginal health board.

Whether run by Indigenous or non-Indigenous people, limited resources—financial and human—hampered health care delivery in Lajamanu. While local control was intended to facilitate choice, the KWCCT was not always given adequate funds to purchase services. Initially, the allocated budget for the various trial health centers was 11 percent less than the actual expenditure of the health centers in the previous year, while "on costs," the cost of employing staff over salaries, was also allocated at a lower rate than that of government services. Furthermore, Territory Health Services invoiced the KWHB on the basis of a flat monthly charge, rather than on a per service basis (Katherine West Health Board 2003, 86). Consequently, purchasing services, particularly from non-governmental vendors, proved cost-prohibitive. During the trial, health centers exceeded the funds supplied by 25.5 percent and financial disputes between the KWHB and THS were common (d'Abbs et al. 2000, 44; Katherine West Health Board 2003, 109). Given the remote location and low population of Aboriginal communities like Lajamanu, health care services were simply more expensive.

The KWHB continued to have difficulties providing a range of services despite eventually receiving greater levels of funding. Due to the high costs of service delivery to areas located hundreds of kilometers from urban centers, there was not enough of a market to motivate the creation of competing providers. In many cases, non-governmental suppliers were nonexistent. Consequently, the Northern Territory government held a virtual monopoly on health care in the bush. In more urban areas, such as Darwin, Alice Springs, and Katherine, it was possible for other providers to emerge; in a remote location such as Lajamanu, this was much more difficult. With the creation of the Katherine West Health Board, it quickly became apparent that the Northern Territory government was, and probably would remain, the only organization that could supply reasonably affordable health care to the region. Government agencies staffed by non-Aboriginal personnel continued to shoulder most of the responsibility because of the limited amount of private enterprise or Aboriginal-owned services in the bush.

When contracting with THS many of the limitations and shortages that the Lajamanu clinic had experienced under government control continued during the trial. While funds were allocated to triple the duration of dentist visits, THS was ultimately unable to deliver the promised service increases, in part because the architect of the initiative had left the Northern Territory (d'Abbs et al. 2000, 55). Territory Health Services was also incapable of achieving goals to increase the number and length of visits by nutritionists, environmental health workers, women's health specialists, and hearing services. The trial evaluators note that

> the experiences of KWHB and THS throughout the Live Phase indicate that extra funding, while a *necessary* condition, is not always a *sufficient* condition for improved services. Difficulties encountered in increasing DMO and dental services, for example, suggest that in an isolated, remote region such as Katherine West, there simply may not be the suitably qualified people and services available for purchase. To the extent that this is so, no amount of restructuring purchaser-provider-funder arrangements will overcome the problem. (d'Abbs et al. 2000, 56)

In spite of establishing an Aboriginal board and increased funding, government services were, for all practical purposes, the only ones available. This situation continues today.

The inability to purchase adequate services can best be demonstrated in the employment of additional full-time staff. As a result of the trial, Lajamanu was given new housing for medical personnel and a resident doctor. While the doctor was a great asset to the community, there were periods when it was impossible to locate a physician willing to work outside of an urban centre. At the beginning of 2009, the clinic was once again without a doctor and relied on regular visits from a physician based in Katherine. When I spoke to Carl about the situation he complained that, even when a doctor was in residence, he or she seldom stayed longer than six months before resigning. The clinic also continues to experience difficulty in hiring and retaining nursing staff. I was told one nurse stepped off the plane, took one look at the community, then turned around and flew back to town. Obtaining additional monies to increase the number of medical positions is of little benefit if personnel choose employment elsewhere.

Whereas the budget for funds allocated to nursing and operational costs were exceeded during the trial, there was a surplus of monies for Aboriginal Health Workers. Of all of the health centers participating in the trail, Lajamanu had the greatest excess: only A\$21,684 was spent out of a budget of A\$99,000 (d'Abbs et al. 2000, 46). This reflects the lack of interest many Aboriginal Health Workers had in remaining employed at the local clinic. Although the promise of community control motivated some Aboriginal Health Workers to go back to work initially, after a short period many became disillusioned at the lack of substantial changes in the clinic environment. The trial evaluators write, "For some months in 1999, a number of Aboriginal Health Workers, particularly in Lajamanu, returned to work in the health centers. However, at the end of 1999 very few of these Aboriginal Health Workers remained in their positions in Lajamanu, partly, it would appear, because of continuing high turnover of nursing staff in that community." (d'Abbs et al. 2000, 53) Once again, it was difficult to translate this money into staff, despite the availability of funding. This situation seems to be continuing. A Warlpiri man informed me that Lajamanu residents still "don't want to work for cheeky nurses."

While community control was intended to give Aboriginal people the power to fire aggressive or incompatible nurses, this did not occur in Lajamanu. Due to an acute staff shortage in remote communities, it was difficult to find replacements for dismissed nurses. Consequently, nurses continued to be employed regardless of their behavior. More than ten years after the introduction of community control, staff in Lajamanu remark that the KWHB is unable to reduce confrontations between nurses and Aboriginal patients significantly. When a serious conflict occurred, the nurse involved was simply moved from one clinic to another. Caroline revealed that after a fellow nurse pushed an Aboriginal patient, the KWHB did not dismiss the perpetrator, but rather transferred her to another location within Katherine West. Caroline added that the KWHB's commitment to ensuring accountable care was a "disappointment."

The constraints of funding, staff, and distance also impacted the design and delivery of new care models intended to acknowledge Aboriginal norms and values. Part of the task of improving the medical services for the communities participating in the trial fell to Roy, a medical advisor for the KWHB. A non-Aboriginal physician who had spent several years treating Aboriginal patients in the Northern Territory, Roy was to act as a liaison between the cultural needs of Lajamanu residents and the clinical needs of the nurses. He was responsible, in part, for recommending a health care model that allowed for greater Aboriginal input and control as well as ensuring that this blueprint also respected clinical protocols. Roy visited Lajamanu every few months in an effort to gather data, conduct interviews, and observe clinical practice in the community. In an attempt to disseminate information about the trial and canvass the opinion of Warlpiri people regarding health care, Roy was often seen working in the clinic or walking around the community.

Roy attempted to address issues brought to his attention but limited funding and lack of staff constrained outcomes. For instance, Sam, an elderly male suffering from a toothache, told Roy that he was reluctant to be examined by the "cheeky" nurses. As an alternative to attending the clinic, Roy agreed to inspect the tooth himself. Once the examination was completed, Roy advised Sam to attend the clinic for treatment, as antibiotics would be necessary to reduce the infection. When Sam hesitated, Roy told him that there was no place else for him to go. This elicited a strong objection from Sam. He said that the clinic had been "useless for a long time now," and expressed frustration that it was "not good for men at all." Sam thought that the clinic should be "a place for all *yapa*" regardless of gender. Roy promised Sam that he would endeavor to make the clinic a more acceptable treatment location for men. Despite this pledge, few changes have occurred. There is a men's exam room in the clinic, but lack of funding and architectural difficulties prohibited the construction of a men's entrance or men's waiting area. Due to gender disparities in nursing, non-Aboriginal staff continue to be predominately female. Given the material conditions in remote communities such as Lajamanu, precipitating major changes in health care delivery was difficult.

Despite these limitations Roy felt that other modifications could be facilitated to improve the cultural appropriateness of the clinic. He believed the ideal method of achieving acceptable health service was through employing *ngangkari* as members of the clinic staff, as well as providing a large supply of bush medicine in the clinic. Once again, there were difficulties in realizing these goals. Since all of the *ngangkari* in Lajamanu were male, it was unlikely that they would have agreed to work within a health center that was so heavily dominated by women. Furthermore, Warlpiri people preferred to consult *ngangkari* well away from the clinic because they knew that the nursing staff generally objected to these practices. Although Roy's plan may at first seem to be a positive step forward, it is fraught with difficulties. Roy simply assumed that culturally appropriate care would be realized by increasing the presence of Warlpiri people in the clinic. As far as I was aware, Roy never asked any Lajamanu residents if they agreed with his assessment.

Although Roy wished to transform the clinic into a more socially acceptable location for treatment, he was unaware of many aspects of Warlpiri social life. After speaking to Sam, Roy commented that he was surprised that the clinic would provoke such a negative reaction. While

Roy eventually became knowledgeable about responses to the clinic, he learned very little about Warlpiri beliefs regarding illness and the body. He believed that Warlpiri people conceived of nurses and *ngangkari* as treating the same diseases, just in different ways. When I mentioned that a *ngangkari* would not attempt to treat diabetes, he expressed surprise. Roy was also ignorant of the notional division between spiritual and physical illnesses, as well as their differing etiologies and treatments. Consequently, non-Aboriginal assumptions regarding Warlpiri beliefs also constrained outcomes.

Roy's lack of knowledge can be attributed to a number of factors. Funding restrictions and the wide range of communities encompassed by the trial limited the amount of time he could spend in Lajamanu. Although he visited the community regularly, Roy had little opportunity to conduct in-depth interviews, let alone develop personal relationships. Like many other visiting medical professionals, he seldom spent more than two days at a time in Lajamanu. Furthermore, the Katherine West Health Board region encompasses a multiethnic area that includes Ngarinman, Ngaliwwuru, Bilinari, Miriuwung-Gadjerong, Warlpiri, Gurindji, Wuli, Mudbara, and Wardaman peoples. There are important differences in term of language, land tenure, and contact history between these groups. Despite this diversity, Roy tended to reify and homogenize many Aboriginal beliefs and practices, such as those concerned with customary prohibitions, *ngangkari*, and bush medicines. Consequently, conventional ideas regarding Aboriginal "culture" were almost universally utilized, while little attention was paid to the actual behaviors of Aboriginal people.

Despite Roy's genuine desire to understand the beliefs and perceptions of Warlpiri people, conversations with Lajamanu residents could focus on public dialogues of Aboriginal irresponsibility and white control, while missing private conversations. With his wife Martha by his side, Larry explained to Roy that an old man had been turned away and verbally abused by the nurses when attempting to seek treatment from the clinic after hours. This type of situation, Larry reported, happened too often: Warlpiri people were not being treated with respect by the nursing staff. He hoped that the Katherine West Health Board would be able to change this situation. But before Larry could explain his opinions in greater detail, Roy cut him off. Roy stated that too often people came to the clinic at midnight with nothing more than a scratch. These "Panadol callouts," he said, were an unnecessary burden on the nursing staff and had to stop. As Roy began to recount the problems facing nurses, Larry's wife Martha communicated to me, through whispers and sign language,[5] that Sarah had been ensorcelled by her father-in-law and was now consulting *ngangkari*.

Later that day, I spoke to Roy and Larry separately about this interaction. Roy commented that actions like noncompliance and late presentation were an indication of a dependence on the health service and non-Aboriginal workers. He wanted people like Larry to realize that these types of behavior had to stop. Concerned primarily with the clinical conduct of Lajamanu residents and possessing little information regarding Warlpiri beliefs of spiritual illness, Roy was oblivious that a conversation about sorcery had been occurring while he complained about late night callouts. In fact, Roy's ignorance of this, and other conversations, allowed him to function as a cultural advocate in Lajamanu. As Lea (2008, 178-179) notes, "It is through *not knowing* the quotidian detail of Aboriginal life, through not knowing the mundane micro-politics of sorcery and such like, *through distance* that we can maintain our claim to cultural sensitively and ethnographic authority." Meanwhile, Larry had a very different response. He asserted that Roy supported the nurses because he was white. Larry believed that racial allegiances and prejudices continued to take precedence over a desire to provide adequate treatment. Despite the promise of community management and culturally appropriate services, Larry said that genuine Warlpiri control had yet to occur.

Embodied Responsibility

While issues such as funding and the availability of service providers influenced the implementation of Katherine West, these factors were not mentioned when I asked Lajamanu residents their opinion of community control. I need to stress the word "ask." Community control was seldom, if ever, discussed. Whereas conversations about the shop, sorcery, aggressive nurses, and illness symptoms were commonplace, I rarely witnessed a discussion about Katherine West that I did not initiate. I discovered that the most positive comments came from people who had either served on the Health Board or had worked with it. Although a former board member complained of having to undergo unwanted medical procedures, she stated that it was now possible to "check up on nurses" and that the clinic was slowly improving. Despite grievances, there was a general belief that non-Aboriginal medical staff made an important contribution to the clinic. One woman said, "Yes they [Aboriginal Health Workers] are good at the clinic. Really though, I am glad those nurses are there. They are ones I trust. Sometimes maybe *yapa* don't know as much." While nursing staff could be cast as "cheeky," Aboriginal workers were often deemed less reliable and less educated than non-Aboriginal staff.

At the start of the Katherine West Coordinated Care Trial, an Aboriginal Health Worker commented, "It would be nice to have our own health service but no one here is trained. We don't know anything so we can't do it." Often lacking professional qualifications, Warlpiri residents had few opportunities for engagement with, or impact on, the management of the clinic aside from acting as members of the health board or as an Aboriginal Health Worker. The tasks of designing a culturally appropriate health care system, running the clinic, and managing staff in Lajamanu were almost exclusively supervised by non-Aboriginal people. In her examination of alliance-building between Aboriginal and non-Aboriginal people in Tennant Creek, Christen (2009) notes that institutional partnerships offer limited options and opportunities for Aboriginal people. Although self-determination and independence are stated outcomes, in reality Aboriginal people continue to be subject to non-Aboriginal strategies. This was not lost on some the residents of Lajamanu who repeatedly equated community control under the KWBH with government control.

The KWHB certainly resembled the government health department in many ways: both were run from an urban center, both were the product of government involvement, and both employed primarily non-Aboriginal workers in Lajamanu. One woman commented, "They tell us it is *yapa* but it still looks like *kardiya* to me." Despite the promises of community control, many residents asserted that racial inequality was still occurring. An elderly woman noted, "Nothing has changed over there. It is the same like before." Similarly, Margaret asserted, "White people are still in charge." When I reminded her that the Health Board was composed solely of Aboriginal people, Margaret commented that, while Lajamanu was represented, they were outnumbered by members from other communities. She added that, despite Aboriginal control of the management of the Health Board, the day-to-day operation of the clinic remained under non-Aboriginal domination.

Dissatisfaction with Aboriginal controlled clinics was not confined to Lajamanu. Martin criticized the care he occasionally received at an Aboriginal controlled clinic in Katherine, complaining the non-Aboriginal nurses treated him like a child because "They think I am a dumb *yapa.*" He added that even the Aboriginal Health Workers were disrespectful. Martin said, "I told them: This is Indigenous organization so you shouldn't work here if you want to be white." As he described difficulties in obtaining pharmaceuticals and insulin from the Katherine clinic, he repeatedly linked his experiences to racial inequality and white prejudice. For some Lajamanu residents, Aboriginal control on paper equated to *kardiya* control in practice.

Rather than stridently supporting or criticizing Katherine West, most Lajamanu residents were ambivalent. My questions about community control were often met with shrugs or silence. I discovered that most people knew very little about the Katherine West Health Board. Stating that he was unaware of either positive or negative outcomes, Carl added that Katherine West was "confidential." Most people were not particularly concerned about the management arrangements of the clinic. In contrast, non-Aboriginal medical staff who arrived in Lajamanu were acutely aware of Katherine West's goal of empowerment. While waiting at the Alice Springs airport, I met a doctor eagerly anticipating his flight to Lajamanu. Having heard many good things about how Aboriginal people had taken over the health services, the doctor commented that he felt honored to work in a community controlled clinic. Although Katherine West was intended to empower Aboriginal residents of Lajamanu, most were indifferent to what many non-Aboriginal health care professionals saw as a momentous event. Despite being squarely aimed at the Aboriginal population, non-Aboriginal people were far more interested and invested in the process of community control.

Upon first arriving to the community, many doctors and nurses praised the positive move to community control. However, by the time they departed, most were disappointed with the results. Two weeks after meeting the doctor, I saw him standing at the airstrip preparing to return to Alice Springs. I asked if Lajamanu had been what he expected. All the doctor could talk about was the poor health of many of the residents and their lack of interest in the health system. He admitted that Lajamanu was not what he had anticipated, given the promises of community control. This statement was echoed by many of the health professionals with whom I spoke. Nurses in Lajamanu often remarked that Katherine West had not led to real Aboriginal control, input, or joint management. Unlike Warlpiri people who complained that non-Aboriginal people had yet to relinquish control, medical staff tended to blame Aboriginal people for the lack of visible change. A visiting doctor believed that because Aboriginal people had a "welfare mentality"—the result, he said, of a history of government management—Katherine West was, and would continue to be, an ineffective tool for increasing local participation in clinical care. Lack of interest in taking over the clinic was seen to be symptomatic of Aboriginal inaction. Health staff often ask what they can do when Aboriginal people do not help themselves (Heil and Macdonald 2008, 313). Similar to nursing narratives surrounding noncompliance, Aboriginal people were cast as disinterested and irresponsible.

Like other medical professionals with whom I have spoken, Caroline wondered what would motivate Aboriginal people to take substantive action to improve their health and health care services. While we were walking down the road one afternoon, she asked what would occur if "all the white people suddenly disappeared." She queried, "Would they get together and do something?" I replied by asking what, exactly, she meant by "do something." As did others, Caroline equated Aboriginal action with "taking over" the health service by working within it. She presumed that Warlpiri people would want to become managers, making decisions and administering health care within an established hierarchy. I pointed out to Caroline that her conceptualization of action was firmly entrenched in non-Aboriginal ideas of management and suggested that Warlpiri responses to community control could be better understood if they were contextualized within Warlpiri political and social structures.

Warlpiri social hierarchies are situated around age and gender. "Looking after" land and *jukurrpa* is a primary way through which authority is exercised. While Warlpiri people cooperate to maintain relatedness and customary law—for instance, through ceremony—there is no structure through which one individual could exert power or make decisions for an entire community (Dussart 2000; Musharbash 2009; Myers 1986; Poirier 2005). Autonomy constitutes an important aspect of personhood (Heil and Macdonald 2008, 304). Prior to the establishment of sedentary communities, serious disputes would result in the aggrieved individuals leaving and set up camp elsewhere. With the introduction of permanent settlements, accusations of sorcery, assaults, and suicide increased, in part because there were no organizational mechanisms for regulating individual behavior toward the community. Authority is exercised through personal ties and allegiances rather than a formal structure composed of distinct and hierarchical positions. Personal autonomy is so highly valued that, even in a crisis situation, it is seldom violated. When a Lajamanu resident became drunk and attempted to commit suicide by cutting his wrists, community members verbally urged him to get medical care but did not physically restrain him. After refusing to go to the clinic, his path was slowly but deliberately blocked, compelling him to begin walking toward the health center. Eventually he entered the clinic, where the nurses were waiting for him. Despite the severity of his condition, actions were taken that did not directly breach his individual autonomy.

Autonomy, a reluctance to coerce others, and an absence of binding collective authority impact Warlpiri responses to initiatives like community control. Lacking a centralized political mechanism, Lajamanu residents are dissuaded from becoming responsible for the clinic and the services that it offers. Health professionals assumed that Aboriginal complaints regarding the provision of health services would lead to desire to take over and formally manage the clinic. This has not happened, in part, because Warlpiri notions of control did not lead to the same conclusion. While some have cast Aboriginal disinterest as the result of laziness or a reliance on government assistance, there is another explanation. Myers (1985, 115) suggests that Aboriginal people could tactically choose to allow non-Aboriginal people to run health services. He (1986, 280) writes, "The employment of outsiders to assume responsibility for the health service was the mechanism through which they managed to objectify it while preserving their own individual autonomy." Despite the tensions that occur, there are practical advantages to allowing non-Aboriginal control. This is not to deny that social barriers to treatment do exist and that Warlpiri residents would prefer that non-Aboriginal medical staff possess greater understanding of, and tolerance for, Aboriginal behaviors. Nevertheless, in some instances, acting outside of Warlpiri social conventions enables the nursing staff to function as a preferred source of treatment.

When asked if Aboriginal people should play a greater role in the clinic, one man responded that Warlpiri people fought too much among themselves and as a result would not be able to effectively manage a health center. If the clinic were controlled primarily by Warlpiri people, the social fabric of Lajamanu would be significantly impacted. Although non-Aboriginal medical staff are often criticized for their lack of cultural understanding, a clinic staffed by *kardiya* provides a uniform level of service and is less disruptive to community relationships. Due to a lack of social obligations outside of their job, nurses keep regular hours and provide a consistent level of care. While all nursing staff are adopted into the kinship system, the duties and avoidance relationships that these affiliations entail are ignored. Keeping non-Aboriginal health practitioners in the community ensures everyone is looked after at all times. Furthermore, as nursing staff are not long-term residents or Aboriginal, violence against them can be carried out without fear of reprisals from other Warlpiri people. Because non-Aboriginal employees leave the community if they feel that a threat is severe, violence is an effective way of removing individuals. After one nurse departs, it seems as if another seamlessly arrives. While some residents acknowledged that doctors could be in short supply in the bush, these same individuals were often unaware of the difficulties faced by the clinic in finding regular nursing staff. The presence of nurses was generally taken for granted. Upon being told that a nurse had resigned, one woman replied, "There are plenty more *kardiya* where she came from.'

Rather than fostering Warlpiri management of the clinic, the coordinated care trial and subsequent management by the KWHB relieved Lajamanu residents from taking control. Brian commented, "No one in the area was really interested in taking over in their particular community, but the KWHB does that now and takes the headache away from each individual community." From the perspective of many medical professionals, it might seem as if community control has not been realized because Warlpiri people are not managing the clinic. However, these notions of what constitutes action are circumscribed and based on non-Aboriginal models of hierarchy. In fact, Warlpiri reluctance to take over the clinic demonstrates the agency of Indigenous people. Contrary to what many non-Aboriginal health professionals had envisioned, Warlpiri people influenced clinical practice simply by not assuming management of the clinic. This is not to deny that Indigenous people continue to be the subject of chronic governance, but I would suggest that a degree of freedom—albeit the freedom to do nothing—exists within these structures. While empowerment is meant to usher in a new era where Indigenous people can take control of their lives and health services, this is not necessarily the case. Constraining the specific roles that Indigenous people can occupy, for instance as cultural liaisons or board members, these programs narrowly conceptualize action, "doing something," as assuming bureaucratic responsibility.

CHAPTER 7

Closing the Gap

"Isn't anyone doing anything to help?" I am often asked this question when discussing the pervasive ill health of Lajamanu. I invariably reply that improving Indigenous health is a national priority in Australia. As a result, a great deal of money is dedicated to increasing health education, upgrading facilities, and ensuring the provision of care. Over half of the Northern Territory's health budget is spent on Aboriginal people, who comprise approximately one third of the population (Northern Territory Department of Health 2004, 35). In 2008, the Commonwealth government committed to providing A$21.5 million boost to remote area health services in the Northern Territory (Macklin 2008, 17). After quoting these figures, the next questions I usually receive are, "Where does all the money go?" and "Why doesn't it make a difference?" To come to grips with the continuing reality of Aboriginal ill health, it is important to explore past and present government health policies and the assumptions that underlie them.

The gap—a phrase used to characterize divergent health outcomes between Aboriginal and non-Aboriginal Australians—has become a well-known and often invoked slogan. In presenting the rates of Aboriginal ill health across the nation, *The Health and Welfare of Australia's Aboriginal and Torres Strait Islander Peoples* reviews "the burden of disease gap," the "mortality gap," and the "disability gap" (Pink and Allbon 2008, 148, 159). Like most other publications examining illness, it notes, "Wherever possible, data are provided . . . on the differences between Indigenous and non-Indigenous Australians" (Pink and Allbon 2008, xxi). The report repeatedly draws attention to the "stark contrast" between Aboriginal and non-Aboriginal data (Pink and Allbon 2008, 156). Statistics are marshaled to illustrate the disparity in health: The mortality rate for Indigenous people is almost three times that of non-Indigenous people, while Indigenous Australians were 1.3 times more likely to suffer from heart diseases and circulatory problems than non-Indigenous Australians, 3.4 times more likely to contract diabetes, and 10 times more likely to have kidney disease (Pink and Allbon 2008, 151, 104). Statistics such as these have motivated a number of initiatives designed to improve Aboriginal health.

One of the first attempts at a new approach to Aboriginal health, the National Aboriginal Health Strategy (1989), aimed to ensure that Aboriginal people would have the same level of access to health services and facilities as their non-Aboriginal counterparts by 2001 (Thomson and English 1992, 23). To achieve this goal the strategy advocated a primary health care approach employing intersectoral cooperation to facilitate improvements in housing, education, and health care delivery (National Aboriginal Health Strategy Working Party 1989). Cross-cultural awareness—possessing an understanding of Aboriginal culture, lifestyle, and sensibilities—was a primary feature of this method. Although "the task of the state is to equalize the outcomes for Indigenous and non-Indigenous: to make the lines on the graph converge," this has come to include a recognition and preservation of cultural difference (Kowal 2010, 190). Unfortunately, the National Aboriginal Health Strategy did not precipitate a noticeable change in health outcomes and a review committee found little evidence of successful implementation (National Aboriginal Health Strategy Evaluation Committee 1994, 2).[1] Despite a lack of results, recent health policies continue to echo the strategy's goals. Almost twenty years later, the importance of environmental health, health promotion, primary health care, and culturally appropriate services continued to be stressed in policy documents.[2]

To complete the picture of Aboriginal health that I have sketched thus far and provide an explanation for why health has not improved despite numerous initiatives, the goals of policy must be examined beside the social, cultural, economic, political, and experiential contexts of Aboriginal communities. As a comprehensive exploration of Indigenous health policy could easily fill an entire volume, I will confine my analysis to four themes that can found throughout many initiatives across the globe: improving environmental health and infrastructure; developing education programs for Indigenous people; endorsing a holistic approach to health care; and educating non-Indigenous health professionals in a cross-cultural approach. These goals are derived from similar assumptions: While improvements in infrastructure and facilities are needed, these changes are not considered sufficient to substantially reduce rates of illness. Aboriginal people must also modify their behaviors. Consequently, health programs stress the importance of improving hygiene, nutrition, and compliance. For many of these health interventions—including the Northern Territory Emergency Response—culture remains a pervasive and persistent theme (O'Mara 2010).

Although well-intentioned, health policies often reproduce popular notions of Indigeneity and lose sight of the day-to-day experiences of Indigenous people. Neatly quantifying disease and claiming to accurately describe the reality of Aboriginal ill health, statistics naturalize difference and maintain the pervasive "vernacular binaries of whitefellas and blackfellas" (Cowlishaw 2004, 10). Much more than a statistical moniker, the gap is another trope equating Aboriginal identity with disparity. In so doing, statistics create the conditions that they seek to explain. Yet in purporting to present the world as it "is," epidemiological data motivate action. Lea (2008, 119) asks, "Why do "we" know about being healthy? Because "we" are structurally enabled to produce and consume the information; we know about the risks, and in a liberal politic, access to information equates to power to act." The results of these actions—policies and initiatives—exemplify government notions of Indigeneity. Examining the rhetoric and reality of development initiatives in Lesotho, Ferguson (1990) asserts that policy documents homogenize and circumscribe peoples and nations. Countries are portrayed as having geography but not history; government but not politics. In Australia, health policies that attempt to close the gap similarly homogenize Indigenous people, while simultaneously embodying governmental perceptions of citizenship, personhood, and social relations.

Regardless of community control, increased resources, and staff, chronic illness pervades Lajamanu and the clinic continues to operate much as it did when I first arrived in 1996. Decades of Indigenous health policies have yet to make a substantial impact on the everyday well-being of Lajamanu residents. One nurse said, "All of those goals and promises really don't affect what we do here. Policies come and go but things in this clinic really don't change." Warlpiri people agree with this assessment, complaining that while politicians make plans in Darwin and Canberra, they continue to suffer in Lajamanu. Responding to a national discourse of disadvantage in which Aboriginal identity is stigmatized, Warlpiri people embody stereotypes and parody the fears of whites. When Aboriginality is equated with illness, enacting stigma can include being sick. Consequently, illness becomes a form of resistance. Although many policies and initiatives focus on improving Aboriginal perceptions of clinical care though self-determination and culturally appropriate treatment, the significance of a stigmatized Aboriginal identity on health outcomes has yet to be acknowledged.

Economy and Environment

Home to a quarter of the Indigenous population, the remote regions of Australia have the worst health in Australia (d'Abbs 1998, 32; Trewin 2006). The physical location of a community is thought to have a significant impact on the health of its inhabitants. For many remote Aboriginal settlements, long distances and low populations constrain the availability of housing, economic growth, and service provision. Homes are overcrowded, people are unemployed, and the clinic is dependent on non-Aboriginal personnel. It is widely accepted that these factors must be addressed if changes in health are to be realized. In an effort to reduce illness rates by enhancing living conditions, a series of health initiatives has been released. Priorities include increasing Aboriginal employment, upgrading resources available to medical service providers, and improving environmental health.[3] While seeking to address what are perceived to be the material and cultural determinants of health, many underlying structural factors have yet to be comprehensively addressed. Instead, health initiatives create a narrative through which notions of remoteness, economy, and Aboriginality are constructed and deployed.

The economic constraints of remote Aboriginal communities are thought to exert a significant impact on health. Poverty, job insecurity, and unemployment have been linked to high rates of morbidity and mortality (Northern Territory Department of Health 2005, 17). Aboriginal jobless rates in the Northern Territory are estimated to be between 53 percent and 57 percent (Northern Territory Department of Health 2005, 24).[4] Low levels of personal income make purchasing food and other essential items difficult. Because Lajamanu is located approximately 600 kilometers from Katherine, transporting foods—particularly fresh fruits and vegetables—is costly and this expense is passed on to consumers. Given the high price of food and low income of many residents, families often ran out of supplies before receiving their fortnightly pay. Socio-economic hardship is believed to be the leading cause of poor nutrition that pervades many Aboriginal communities (Harrison 1991, 163; Humphery, Dixon, and Marrawal 1998, 98).

One way of providing economic development and greater levels of Aboriginal participation in the health care system is to encourage Aboriginal employment. Health discourse and government policy regularly stress the need to make this goal a reality. In its five-year plan, the Northern Territory government notes that Aboriginal employment is a health and service quality issue. It asserts, "Improving both Aboriginal representation in the health workforce and ensuring that they have access to career and development opportunities is an essential component of building a different and better functioning Department." (Northern Territory Department of Health 2005, 37). It hopes to increase Aboriginal representation in the health and community services workforce to 15 percent and expand the roles of Aboriginal personnel.

Regardless of these objectives, a number of barriers prevent Lajamanu residents from obtaining employment in the health service industry. Many Warlpiri people did not possess a high standard of literacy and numeracy skills and were unable or unwilling to enter the workforce. Because of the lack of higher education facilities in the community, students must travel to Batchelor, several hundred kilometers away. Many residents disliked spending so much time separated from their families and were reluctant to undertake further studies. Even if people were trained and, for instance, had attained an Aboriginal Health Worker qualification, they did not always offer themselves for work. Conflicts with the non-Aboriginal medical staff over the use of vehicles and time off regularly acted as a disincentive. Furthermore, Aboriginal Health Workers occasionally had difficulties meeting the expectations of nurses and community residents.

Despite the introduction of community control in Lajamanu, a non-Aboriginal workforce continued to manage the day-to-day operation of the clinic and provide the bulk of medical treatment. However, even non-Aboriginal workers were in short supply. Positions were often filled by temporary staff or remained open. In addition, there was a high turnover of medical personnel. Without the continuity of long-term staff, it was difficult to establish good relationships with community members and tailor health care services to meet their needs. Tellingly, low rates of retention were often blamed on conflicts with Aboriginal people and subsequent burnout. Examining the Territory Health Service, Lea (2008, 189) notes, "The equation—remote area work is beset with difficulties which lead to burnout, which leads to high turnover—has solidified into a commonplace. Meanwhile, on the rare occasions when it is noted, the high turnover that is equally, if not more, true of senior management positions in central office locations is ascribed to the corporatized need for managers to constantly replenish their careers, to refuse stagnation by frequently reinventing themselves." While job turnover was uniformly high throughout the Northern Territory, nursing rates were rationalized by invoking remoteness, stress, and the difficulties of adjusting to life in Aboriginal communities. Staffing narratives mirror wider tendencies to invoke the exceptionalism of remote areas and the Aboriginal people that inhabit them.

One of the most visible issues raised when discussing the continued ill health of Aboriginal people is housing. In a recent budget report, the Commonwealth government notes, "the poorest housing and greatest housing need is undoubtedly in remote communities. Here, overcrowded and sub-standard housing is the norm. Isolation and climate make houses difficult and expensive to build. They wear out quickly" (Macklin 2008, 11). In many communities such as Lajamanu, all of the homes in the community are owned and managed by an Indigenous housing organization, which receives most of its funding through government grants. However, these organizations are chronically under resourced and homes are in poor repair. It is estimated that 70 percent of Aboriginal homes in remote Northern Territory communities have major structural problems (Australian Bureau of Statistics 2002, table 1) and 61 percent are overcrowded (Pink and Allbon 2008, 41). There are an average of 4.7 people per home, although as many as 33 have been recorded (Bailie and Wayte 2006, 179). In Lajamanu, the acute housing shortage resulted in several extended family members inhabiting a single home. It was not unusual to have ten to fifteen people living in a three-bedroom house.

Most Lajamanu homes were not well-maintained or kept in a sanitary condition. I was told that, with so many people living together, there was little point in cleaning. In a short time, a tidy home would be dirtied by residents, visitors, or animals. Front doors seldom latched properly, allowing dogs to have free access to any food lying around. White walls were sometimes covered with brown spots, the result of food that had been thrown by children. In one house, the refrigerator was infested with dozens of cockroaches. Opening the door sent them scurrying for cover into an open bag of bread. Bedding, dishes, cups, and utensils were frequently shared and seldom cleaned. Toilets were not consistently flushed or sanitized. Consequently, the condition of Aboriginal residences has been recognized as an important factor impacting high rates of poor health.

Medical staff and researchers note that lack of sanitation encourages a variety of bacterial strains to thrive, skin diseases such as scabies to spread, and gastrointestinal complaints to flourish.[5] Bailie and Runcie (2001, 364) report that "The poor state of housing and access to adequate facilities for washing have been identified as key underlying factors in the high levels of morbidity and mortality from bacterial respiratory tract infections and the significant contribution of such infections to the generally poor state of health of many Indigenous Australians." Recurrent bacterial infections exacerbate pre-existing chronic diseases. Although tuberculosis has been eliminated in most of Australia, it continues to plague some remote Aboriginal communities, in part, because of constant overcrowding. In addition to encouraging infectious and chronic disease, crowded homes also intensify the effects of smoking and are thought to contribute to domestic violence (Board of Inquiry into the Protection of Aboriginal Children from Sexual Abuse 2007).

As calls for better resources are answered by building additional housing in Lajamanu, new homes quickly decay and come to resemble existing structures. The inability to maintain homes and ensure domestic hygiene has been alternately blamed on a racist state (Morgan 2006) and a lack of consultation with Aboriginal homeowners (Lee and Morris 2005). However, the most popular explanation implicates the behavior of Aboriginal people (Hughes 2007; Sutton 2009). As Lea and Pholeros (2010, 189) note, "The prevailing theory is that houses become structurally compromised in swift time frames more or less because of the way householders tend the house." But examining the materials and construction specifications of Aboriginal community housing has led them to assert that, contrary to the popular view of Aboriginal irresponsibility, it is the home itself that is often to blame. While these structures might have the appearance of homes found elsewhere in Australia, in reality they are shoddily built with substandard hardware. Lea and Pholeros (2010, 197) add that in assessing home maintenance and hygiene, researchers often employ surveys that are not standardized, allow for only yes or no responses, and spend little time (if any) inspecting the home or speaking to residents. Although statistics are marshaled to present a "real" account of Aboriginal housing, they are nonetheless employed strategically.

Examining a cholera epidemic in Venezuela, Briggs and Mantini-Briggs (2003) found that citizenship was similarly articulated through notions of health and sanitation. Being deemed "unsanitary" subjects—failing to accept medical notions of hygiene and compliance—profoundly affected Indigenous people's access to the "political, social, and civil dimensions of citizenship," including health care (Briggs and Mantini-Briggs 2003, 11). A "meta-narrative of blame" was created in which remoteness became naturalized (Briggs and Mantini-Briggs 2003, 215). Rather than examining the social processes that generated and perpetuated the label of remoteness, geographic isolation and cultural difference were blamed for the lack of service provision and economic development. As a result, the health messages of the epidemic actually increased racism against Indigenous people while their health conditions worsened.

A similar situation is occurring in Australia. Remoteness has become naturalized, pathologized, and associated with Aboriginality. Rather than looking at the goals of settlement—to create Aboriginal communities close to cattle stations but distant from white towns—remoteness is seen to be a consequence of geography, not social engineering. Remote communities then become known for having the worst health, highest rates of violence against nursing staff, poorest living conditions, and highest adherence to "culture." These views are bolstered by statistics that are presented as scientific, unbiased, and self-evident. Sutton (2009, 74) asserts that it is only through statistical data that we can truly know if Aboriginal health is improving. He fails to acknowledge the social meanings and discursive force that have become embedded in this data. Repeatedly blaming high rates of nursing turnover on poor living conditions, stress, and violence, will likely dissuade many nurses from accepting positions in remote communities. Attributing poor health to overcrowded and unhygienic homes and then holding Aboriginal residents responsible lead to neoliberal views that advocate encouraging the abandonment of Aboriginal practices. In seeking to represent the reality of life in Aboriginal communities, statistical narratives perpetuate inequality. Portrayed as "facts," these assumptions have serious consequences for government policies, service provision, and, ultimately, the lives of Aboriginal people.

Health Education

The everyday actions of Aboriginal people are considered to be a major barrier to improved health. High rates of morbidity and mortality are regularly attributed to behavioral factors such as poor hygiene, eating habits, and pharmaceutical noncompliance (Pink and Allbon 2008; Stewart 1997; Northern Territory Department of Health 1998b). The assumption often made by government and health care professionals is "If only Aboriginal people understood the true import of the alarming data that professionals have to hand, they would readily commit to appropriate lifestyle changes" (Lea 2008, 119). To precipitate these changes many health initiatives and policies focus on teaching Aboriginal people to adopt healthier "habits." The Northern Territory government (1997, 18) notes, "Access to modern health facilities and expert medical attention will not on its own overcome the poor health standard of Aboriginal people, if they are not also linked to a greater awareness of health issues through sound education programs." In its five-year plan, the Northern Territory was especially committed to providing sexual education for adolescents and nutritional education for pregnant women (Northern Territory Department of Health 2005). It is hoped that once individuals are made aware of the benefits of improved nutrition and compliance, they will alter their behavior.

In Lajamanu, health education messages were found throughout the community, including the store, clinic, and school. One of the clinic walls was lined with books and pamphlets designed to educate individuals about diet, sanitation, and other topics. All were written in simple English and contained numerous photos and illustrations. For instance, *The Toilet Book* discusses the importance of flushing and keeping the toilet clean, while several others were devoted to imparting an understanding of diabetes and the dangers of eating foods high in fat and sugar. But health messages were not only confined to the clinic. At the store, signs declared "Bush Foods Are Best." An illustrated chart of the food groups once hung over the entrance to the shop. It not only included sugar and flour but also kangaroo, bush honey, and witchetty grubs. In the Lajamanu Community Council office, a poster featuring an Aboriginal "Condom Man" was displayed in an effort to encourage safe sex. In addition to visual messages, medical staff constantly reminded patients to eat nutritious foods, take their pills, and attend the clinic in a timely manner. Almost every day Lajamanu residents were confronted by health education messages in one form or another.

Health education strategies have been effective in the sense that Lajamanu residents are aware of many of the health issues that impact their lives. Medical staff and educational materials have successfully taught the importance of nutrition, exercise, and the management of chronic disease. Diabetics were well-informed about the causes and treatment for their illness, often reporting that an ideal treatment regime consisted of avoiding sugars and taking pharmaceuticals. Many residents were able to break down foods into those with protein, carbohydrates, and sugars but this knowledge has not motivated them to alter pre-existing eating patterns. In many cases, adopting medical ideas did not lead to a substantial change in health behavior. Urging people to eat a healthier diet one man said, "You go up to the shop and buy all that greasy food. Chips, chicken wings, meat pies. All of that is rubbish. It is high in fat and stops this one [points to chest]." Regardless of this statement, he often purchased food from the takeaway. Although Lajamanu residents were exposed to a great many messages about the importance of nutrition and most individuals vowed to consume healthy meals, it did not prevent these same individuals from continuing to eat foods high in sugar and fat. Diabetics discussed the dangers of sugar while spooning it into their tea.

Education initiatives forget that the relationship between knowledge and action is complex. Possessing abstract notions of illness and its treatment does not guarantee that these ideas will be followed in practice.[6] The choices that people make are motivated by a number of variables, not only knowledge. Throughout this book I have demonstrated that, while Warlpiri people hold notions about their bodies, health and illness, these notions tend to play less of a role in health behavior than factors such as poverty, social concerns, and experience.

Being able to recognize that something was "wrong" is an important first step to seeking treatment. Because many people were accustomed to experiencing aches and pains as a routine element of everyday life, mild headaches, fatigue, and occasional gastrointestinal complaints were rarely identified as requiring much, if any, care. It was only after symptoms became more acute that individuals would contemplate seeking treatment, such as taking prescription medication. While the skin irritation of scabies motivated the application of pharmaceutical ointments, prescription medication to control diabetes was utilized infrequently, in part, because few members of the community could distinguish symptoms. Despite the information and test results provided by the medical staff, a clinical treatment regime was seldom followed. Without the feeling of being sick, there was little motivation to change behavior, particularly in a socially and economically circumscribed environment such as Lajamanu. Consequently, everyday experience generally determined health behavior much more than an abstract knowledge of disease.

In addition to experience, the economic environment of the community constrained actions. Whether purchasing food from the takeaway or hunting kangaroos, individuals needed access to cash. Economic realities, such as low incomes, fortnightly pay periods, and high food prices, dictated when and what kinds of food were bought and consumed. While many people enjoyed eating apples and were aware that fresh fruits provided a valuable source of nutrition, produce tended to be significantly more expensive than processed foods. Consequently, knowledge of nutrition and an enjoyment of apples did not automatically result in an increased consumption of fruit. Similarly, the economic realities of community life limited hunting and gathering activities. The costs of a sturdy vehicle, petrol, gun, and bullets were substantial when compared to the small amount of food that would be procured.

Warlpiri people also navigated a social environment in which conventions surrounding generosity and gender structured many interactions. A great deal of reciprocity occurred through demand sharing, in which the redistribution of resources created and maintained social relationships. Expensive and sought-after foods, such as apples, were particularly subject to demands. After arriving in the community I became accustomed to children appearing at my door and insisting, "Give me apple." In an attempt to avoid losing food to hungry kin, individuals employed a number of practical strategies such as keeping shopping trips to a minimum and concealing food. One particularly effective tactic was purchasing prepared food from the takeaway. Prepared food was relatively inexpensive, did not need to be stored, and could be easily concealed. Although people were well aware that takeaway food was generally less nutritious than other options, the considerations of everyday life took precedence over health education messages.

While norms of reciprocity influenced food consumption, norms regulating gender and family relations similarly impacted rates of clinical consultations. Lajamanu residents preferred to obtain treatment from members of the same gender or close kin. As most of the medical staff were non-Aboriginal and female, Warlpiri women attended the clinic in larger numbers. In contrast, men were often reluctant to seek medical treatment. The social discomfort of shame could outweigh the physical discomfort of illness. Relationships between Aboriginal Health Workers and residents also impacted treatment strategies. Kinship avoidance relations could deter sick individuals from entering the clinic, while having family members working as Aboriginal Health Workers could encourage repeated visits. Seeking treatment at the clinic was a social encounter. As a result, avoiding the clinic did not necessarily entail avoiding biomedical therapies. Even if the clinic was not consulted, individuals would utilize medication or other biomedical technologies independently. As an illness became more severe the likelihood of consulting the nurses or Aboriginal Health Workers increased. When serious illnesses were left untreated and allowed to reach an advanced stage, it was most often the result of attempts to avoid shame, not avoid biomedical treatment.

Experience, norms, and economy significantly impacted the choices of Lajamanu residents. However, when recounting a tale of clinical treatment, postulating the cause of a health crisis, or providing health advice to others, these factors often took a back seat to generalized physiological, cosmological, or etiological beliefs. Warlpiri people possess a comprehensive cosmology and often use these concepts when explaining a therapeutic regimen. For example, a male could justify a reluctance to seek biomedical treatment by claiming to be ensorcelled, a condition that the clinic was considered unable to effectively cure. Despite such a statement, gender norms also provided a disincentive to visit the clinic. In addition to notions regarding sorcery and spiritual illness, Warlpiri people are accustomed to discussing nutrition, physiology, and genetics. In these instances, a similar pattern occurred. I heard statements praising bush foods as a source of nutrition far more often than those regarding the economic difficulties of hunting and gathering.

While an individual's motivations are multifaceted, narratives are employed to make public sense of past events and justify responses to them within existing social constraints. In Lajamanu, illness was a personal problem and a topic of community interest. Talk about health permeated card games, interactions at the shop, and telephone conversations. Disease was not just a physical event; it was a social one. Consequently, illness narratives expressed medical ideas as well as social sentiments. Tales of sorcery, genetically inherited disease, nutritious bush meat, or ineffective pharmaceuticals commented upon relationships between individuals and groups. An accusation of sorcery could be tied to an incident of domestic violence, while an alternative diagnosis of genetic abnormalities could contest this claim. Relationships were embodied through contrasting etiologies. These illness explanations were also social explanations.

Although medical beliefs are used to make sense of actions, these beliefs are not the sole determinant of behavior. Individuals approach illness at specific moments and under specific circumstances. While it is possible to ground an analysis in past episodes, there is no predictable roadmap that is universally followed. Notions regarding the inability of biomedicine to treat spiritual illness or the nutritional benefits of hunting and gathering did not predict actual conduct. In reality, asserting that an illness was the result of sorcery did not preclude clinical explanations or treatment. Consequently, the continued belief in sorcery should not be seen as a threat to biomedical treatment. If a patient delays in consulting the clinic, it is probably because of norms, familiarity, and convenience, more than an adherence to Warlpiri cosmology concerning spiritual illness. Similarly, accepting biomedical protocols did not always encourage greater rates of pharmaceutical use. Vowing to eat bush food for health benefits did lead to hunting and gathering. *Ngangkari*, nurses, pharmaceuticals and bush medicines were used as options that may or may not be the most comfortable, accessible, socially acceptable, or expedient way to end disease. The goals of policy are difficult to achieve, in part, because Warlpiri health behavior is entrenched in the practical environment of the community as well as the experience of illness.

Holistic Health

Throughout Australia, notions of, and responses to, Aboriginal culture suffuse medical service provision and act as a lynchpin in the delivery of primary health care. Referred to as "the key to improving health," primary health care seeks to provide culturally appropriate medical care for Aboriginal people (Public Accounts Committee 1996, 32). The National Aboriginal Health Strategy (National Aboriginal Health Strategy Working Party 1989, x) defines primary health care as "Essential health care based on practical, scientifically sound, socially and culturally acceptable method, and technology made universally accessible to individuals and families in the communities in which they live through their full participation at every stage of development in the spirit of self-reliance and self-determination." Primary health care attempts to move from a medical model to a curative one, shifting the focus from episodic disease treatment to continuous health maintenance. Nevertheless, treatment still takes place through biomedical facilities, such as the clinic and hospital. Effective primary health care providers should arrest the disease in an appropriate and effective manner, while acknowledging the way in which Aboriginal people conceive of wellness. Today, primary health care is strongly endorsed by the Northern Territory Department of Health and Families (Northern Territory Department of Health 2005; 2008a). To further contextualize health initiatives, it is necessary to examine the origins of primary health care, its assumptions, and implementation.

Primary health care was born out of the World Health Organization (WHO) and its holistic definition of health. Although international medical cooperation existed prior to World War II, it was the subsequent formation of the WHO that ushered in a new era of global initiatives. Founded by a generation of social medicine physicians, the WHO sought to understand the social and economic factors of illness, while providing care for all members of society (Brady, Kunitz, and Nash 1997). As a result, a new definition of health was adopted in 1946, "a state of complete mental and social well-being and not merely the absence of disease or infirmity" (World Health Organization 1946). Health was no longer simply a lack of bodily symptoms; it required personal, social, and physical well-being. The WHO definition would come to exert a profound impact on conceptions of Aboriginal health within Australia as well as on the strategies intended to improve morbidity and mortality.

More than two decades after the WHO reconceptualized the definition of health, the well-being of Australia's Aboriginal people was thrust into the national spotlight. By the 1970s, increasing calls for Aboriginal rights to land and social equality transformed health into a key political issue. As a result, demands for self-determination and independent health services increased. In 1971, the first community controlled clinic began operation, setting a precedent that would be repeated across the nation. Aboriginal rights advocates and supporters of community control seized on the WHO definition of health. Utilizing international perspectives, Aboriginal health was transformed from a local state issue to one of national importance. Brady, Kunitz, and Nash (1997, 278) write, "By embracing the Alma Ata principles of primary health care and the broad definition of health, Aboriginal organizations have been able to lobby for ideals of social justice, equality and access, and fend off suggestions that separate services are a luxury that the government cannot afford." Across Australia, the importance of empowerment, community control, and culturally appropriate services was affirmed by invoking the WHO concept of holistic health.

By the 1980s the Commonwealth and Territory governments were asserting that Indigenous conceptions of health were holistic. The National Aboriginal Health Strategy (National Aboriginal Health Strategy Working

Party 1989, ix) comments, "It would be difficult from an Aboriginal perspective to conceptualize 'health' as one aspect of life." The policy stresses that for Aboriginal people health is "not just the physical well-being of the individual but the social, emotional, and cultural well-being of the whole community" (National Aboriginal Health Strategy Working Party 1989, x). These views were endorsed throughout Australia (Maher 1999; Mobbs 1991; Morgan, Slade, and Morgan 1997; Nathan and Leichleitner 1983). Reid (1982, 92) notes, "In many ways, the Aboriginal perspective on health and illness is closer than that of Western medicine to the World Health Organization's definition of health." Medical researchers, health care practitioners, anthropologists, and political advocates almost universally assert that fundamental differences between Aboriginal and biomedical approaches to health exist. Stressing the importance of social harmony for maintaining health, Aboriginal conceptions are contrasted with biomedical ones, which are portrayed as "particularistic, biophysical and mechanistic" (Nathan and Leichleitner 1983, 91). Whereas Aboriginal medicine is concerned with the group, biomedicine rarely transcends the individual.

Notions of holistic Aboriginal health traditions and mechanistic biomedical protocols have been invoked to portray the former as revitalizing and the latter as a means of domination. Since the 1980s, a number of Indigenous and non-Indigenous critiques of biomedical research and service provision have appeared (Humphery 2001). In some cases, calls are made to repudiate biomedicine and its methods. Flick and Nelson (1994, 4) write, "Using western scientific methodology and demanding rigorous empirical evidence of benefit, as defined within this scientific approach, is a continuation of the patronizing practice of imposition." Batchelor College encouraged an understanding of Aboriginal lifestyle choices from a holistic viewpoint in an effort not to repeat the "errors of the last two hundred years" (Grootjans and Spiers 1996, 12). In some settings, calls for self-determination, land rights, and Aboriginal empowerment replaced those for biomedical interventions (Mathews 1996, 30; Mobbs 1991, 301). In these instances, assumptions of conflicting Aboriginal and biomedical traditions are marshaled as a political tool to express and validate demands for Aboriginal rights.

Policies that encourage a separation from, or rejection of, non-Aboriginal methodologies, endorse a break with an assimilationist past but have yet to transcend the categories of this era. Stressing the incommensurability of Aboriginal and biomedical approaches simply replicates previously existing assumptions. Concepts such as holistic health, whether endorsed by the government or Aboriginal health advocates, continue to reify notions of Aboriginality and biomedicine, automatically casting them as conflicting. This is not to deny that differences do exist between Aboriginal and biomedical etiologies and treatment regimens or that medicine has been used as a political tool to constrain the lives of Aboriginal people. However, perspectives emphasizing biomedicine's ill fit within the cultural context of Aboriginal communities have been born out of national and international struggles over meaning, funding, and resources. Conceptualizing biomedical and Aboriginal approaches as fundamentally different, and asserting that the latter is superior to the former because it is holistic, serves to advance arguments for community controlled health services and self-determination. In fact, holism, which is now used to epitomize Indigenous approaches to health in opposition to Western methods, was actually born out of the biomedical ideals of social medicine.

Examining the daily lives of individuals in Lajamanu reveals that the dichotomy between Aboriginal and biomedical etiologies and treatments was not as oppositional as many national health discourses portray. Many researchers tend to equate Aboriginal ideas of health to what Warlpiri people refer to as spiritual illness. However, Lajamanu residents also recognized another class of illness: physical. While spiritual illness affected the soul and was the result of social conflict, physical illness was the outcome of environmental factors like cold weather or viruses. As did doctors and nurses, Aboriginal people also viewed illness as caused by a malfunctioning biological entity, the body. In practice, Warlpiri notions physical illnesses and biomedical etiologies were often conflated. Diabetes, like *minta*, was considered to be a physical illness. Furthermore, diseases like *minta* could be attributed to a heat imbalance or a virus. In Lajamanu, a single etiological system existed; there was no clash. Aboriginal people have incorporated new ideas and technologies into existing beliefs and social practices.

In addition to disease etiologies, treatment behaviors were also integrated. Lajamanu residents took analgesics, went to the clinic, collected bush medicines, and visited *ngangkari*. Although they tended to praise treatments classified as *yapa-kurlangu* over those labeled *kardiya-kurlangu*, this did not deter their use of biomedical technologies. A variety of therapies could be utilized for a single illness episode. Individuals suffering from nasal congestion would sniff bush medicines, take a nasal decongestant, or both. These treatment methods did not fundamentally conflict with one another. Ill individuals were concerned with getting well, not strictly adhering to an Aboriginal or biomedical system. Furthermore, the use of biomedical facilities is heavily influenced by Warlpiri norms and customs. Gender concerns exert a significant impact on rates of presentation and Lajamanu residents can expect Aboriginal Health Workers to observe customary prohibitions in the clinic. As the previous chapter argues, employing non-Aboriginal staff is one way in which Aboriginal people are able to maintain individual autonomy within a health care setting. Consequently, the clinic does not stand apart from the community or its values.

Interpretations of treatment are also integrated. Almost fifty years ago, Cawte and Kidson (1964, 981) described a *ngangkari* who believed a surgical scar was evidence of an attempt to steal his *nguwa*. In this example, the fear of losing *nguwa* to another *ngangkari* during treatment is transferred to a hospital environment. In Lajamanu, Jacob described losing a portion of his *nguwa* as a result of diabetes complications. In each case Aboriginal cosmology intersects biomedical treatments and explanations. The idea of two competing and distinct medical systems that revolve around cosmological or scientific differences must be re-evaluated in light of the day-to-day lives of Lajamanu residents. While a recurrent theme in policy documents is the difference between Indigeneity and biomedicine, Indigenous people practically and efficiently incorporate a range of etiologies and treatments into local settings. Clinical practices and technologies are integrated into Warlpiri lives far more than most health policies assume.

Cross-Cultural Skills

For health care providers, culture remains a prominent theme in understanding the behaviors of Aboriginal people (O'Mara 2010). Non-Indigenous medical professionals have been accused of possessing little knowledge or respect of local beliefs and, as a result, alienating Indigenous clients (Mitchell 2007; Mobbs 1991; Nathan and Leichleitner 1983; National Aboriginal Health Strategy Working Party 1989; Paradies 2007; Public Accounts Committee 1996; Saggers and Gray 1991). In 1994, the National Aboriginal Health Strategy Evaluation advocated the introduction of cultural awareness training programs (National Aboriginal Health Strategy Evaluation Committee 1994, 14). Since that time cultural awareness has become a common theme in Aboriginal health policy. As Lea (2008, 98) notes, "No self-respecting orientation program in a government agency which proclaims Aboriginal issues as part of its core business could fail to specifically cover "working cross-culturally." The Northern Territory's five-year plan for improving Aboriginal health prioritizes the "education of professional and other staff about the importance of Aboriginal culture and values in the delivery of health services" (Northern Territory Department of Health 2005, 27). *Ampe Akelyernemane Meke Mekarle "Little Children Are Sacred"*—the report that precipitated the Northern Territory Emergency Response—states that "an understanding of Aboriginal culture and 'world view' is an essential prerequisite to being able to work with Aboriginal people to achieve successful outcomes" (Board of Inquiry into the Protection of Aboriginal Children from Sexual Abuse 2007, 202). It adds, "basic cultural awareness should be compulsory for all government staff" (Board of Inquiry into the Protection of Aboriginal Children from Sexual Abuse 2007, 202). In 2008, the Northern Territory Department of Health and Families endorsed a new policy of cultural security that was designed to help staff work cross-culturally as part of a primary health care approach to improve health.

Cross-cultural training is intended to increase rates of pharmaceutical use and treatment as well as reduce hostile interactions between Aboriginal people and non-Aboriginal medical personnel. In addition, cultural security is seen as an effective strategy to minimize costs and risk, while increasing market share. The Northern Territory's Department of Health (2005, 26) notes that, outside Australia, some malpractice insurers provide significant discounts to medical personnel who have completed cultural competency training. Looking to the cultural security policy as a money-saving tool, it is hoped that providing better services will reduce rates of noncompliance, which in turn will lower the number of evacuations and recurring consultations. Furthermore, the policy could precipitate lower insurance rates and associated costs. However, the phrase "cross-cultural training" is not well defined and the notion of culture is simply taken for granted. While the cultural competence of non-Aboriginal medical staff remains a crucial aspect of many health initiatives, most policy documents do not give examples of cultural norms or beliefs that non-Aboriginal medical staff will be taught (Heil 2006, 104).

Over the past decade, the Northern Territory government has run a variety of cross-cultural training programs for medical professionals. Some lasted only a day, while others took several to complete. Examining a four-day cross-cultural training course provided by the Territory Health Service (THS), Lea (2008) documents the process through which Aboriginal beliefs and practices become transformed from complex understandings to a series of dot-points on a white board. Anthropological ideas, such as Sansom's assertion that words can be a form of currency, become simplified into admonitions to avoid asking Aboriginal people direct questions (Lea 2008, 82). Employees of THS were taught several concise guidelines to govern their interactions with Aboriginal people, such as, eye contact should be avoided; women should keep their knees covered and refrain from wearing trousers; Aboriginal people will say "yes" to please you; country is important; avoid asking direct questions; and Aboriginal people have a high tolerance for pain (Lea 2008, 98). Lea (2008, 108-109) notes, "There are double enigmas here—kinship connection that are barely comprehended yet understood as powerfully controlling—reminding us again, if we needed reminding, of the mysterious inexplicability of Aboriginal people lurking behind the dot-pointed summaries of their culture. . . ." Rather than imparting a comprehensive understanding of Aboriginal beliefs and practices, the session served to underscore the fundamental difference between Aboriginal and non-Aboriginal people.

At the conclusion of the four-day session, participants were confronted with the reality of violence in Aboriginal communities (Lea 2008, 109). As was the custom at THS, this discussion was conducted around a whiteboard upon which descriptions of violent behavior were written. In this way, violence itself became disembodied and transformed into a series of dot-points. Although not on the official agenda, the session ended with a self-defense class. Lea (2008, 114) sums up the experience, "A total schema for apprehending the frightening space between us and them has been signed, sealed and delivered, with rules for respectful dialogue and lessons in self-defense." In compartmentalizing culture and violence, the training session overlooked the social complexities that underlie interactions between Aboriginal and non-Aboriginal people. Cultural awareness programs, such as the those offered by THS, have been routinely criticized for failing to acknowledge the power differentials that structure race relationships in health care settings, including the pervasive reality of structural violence (Jenks 2011; Kleinman and Benson 2006a; Rouse 2010; Shaw and Armin 2011).

In addition to completing cross-cultural training courses, some members of the non-Aboriginal medical staff have been working in Aboriginal

communities for years. Through their own initiative, a few have suc-
ceeded in learning a great deal about Aboriginal people. For instance,
Sharon took pride in being a nurse who was aware of Aboriginal beliefs
regarding spiritual illness. Prior to coming to Lajamanu, she had served in
Aboriginal communities throughout the Northern Territory and Western
Australia. Sharon stated that *ngangkari* were simply another form of treatment that should be utilized if biomedical options failed or were incon-
clusive. If patients were suffering from pain or fever and she was unable
to "find anything wrong with them," Sharon recommended consulting a
ngangkari. Sharon said there were occasions when she told patients there
was nothing she could do medically and then sent them directly from
the clinic to see *ngangkari*. However, if medical practitioners were able to
identify an illness or pathogen, Sharon felt that clinical treatment was the
only effective option. When Sarah began consulting *ngangkari* after being diagnosed with SLE, Sharon replied that she was "wasting her time."
Medical tests clearly indicated that Sarah was not suffering from the effects of sorcery.

I spoke with very few non-Aboriginal medical professionals who "believed" in *ngangkari* and Sharon was the only nurse who admitted to referring patients to them. No doubt Sharon's behavior was not what the
Northern Territory government envisioned when they stressed the importance of cross-cultural training. Nevertheless, it raises a number of issues.
On one hand, Sharon could be seen as respecting Aboriginal beliefs by
endorsing the utilization of biomedical and Aboriginal forms of treatment as well as acknowledging the role of *ngangkari* in Aboriginal communities. Perhaps if Lajamanu residents believed that they could speak
openly to a nurse about their fears of sorcery, it might encourage them
to come to the clinic sooner, thereby increasing rates of biomedical treatment. On the other hand, some health professionals might respond that
by sending people to *ngangkari*, Sharon is actually discouraging clinical
forms of treatment and perhaps increasing late presentation. Examining
Sharon's tenure in Lajamanu illustrates the way in which medical treatment can be affected when a member of the nursing staff expressed a belief in spiritual illness.

Interestingly, sending some ill individuals to consult *ngangkari* did
not seem to encourage or discourage presentation at the clinic. During
Sharon's stay in Lajamanu, the clinic functioned much as it always had.
Regardless of her belief in sorcery, Sharon's attitude and behavior were
similar to that of many of the other nurses. She often complained that

Aboriginal people were chronically irresponsible. If she felt that patients were "being difficult" or "not acting responsibly," Sharon scolded them, commenting "they don't want to hear that." She firmly believed that certain protocols must be followed and patients should take their medication regularly and on time. Sharon readily acknowledged that many of her interactions with Aboriginal people ended in conflict and joked about the number of irate Aboriginal patients that she had dealt with over the years. As noted in Chapter 5, Sharon once exclaimed, "My skin name is white cunt!"

Cross-cultural awareness is supposed to lead to friendlier interactions between medical staff and Aboriginal patients, but in Lajamanu this was not the case. Despite possessing an understanding of Aboriginal beliefs, Sharon could engage in bitter arguments with Warlpiri people. Sharon's presence in the clinic did not change the circumstances of treatment. A belief in the abilities of *ngangkari* did not produce an acceptance of Aboriginal health behaviors. Similarly, Dorothy was aware of Aboriginal naming norms, but she also scolded people for not complying with medication or unnecessarily calling her out after hours. A nurse might understand a bit about Warlpiri cosmology and customs but this did not inevitably translate into a greater acceptance of Warlpiri health behavior, particularly when that behavior that was considered to pose health risks. Regardless of their differing knowledge, nursing staff almost uniformly asserted that Aboriginal people could be irresponsible and, as a result, admonished patients for failing to seek clinical treatment in a timely manner or take their medication appropriately.

Although an emphasis has been placed on the existence of cultural education programs for non-Aboriginal medical staff, such courses might do little to reduce hostile interactions in the clinic. With diagnosis and treatment occupying the majority of their time, nurses are firmly oriented toward biomedical health outcomes (Ritchie 2001). When Lajamanu residents, for whatever reason, disregarded medical guidelines, nurses became frustrated. Actions that nurses believed impacted health negatively were stridently discouraged. As long as patients continued to engage in "detrimental" conduct, nurses saw little reason to change their attitudes toward Warlpiri people. Knowledge of Aboriginal beliefs—much like knowledge of nutrition or diabetes—was only one of several factors that guided action. Like health education campaigns, cross-cultural training initiatives tend to overlook the role of experience while reifying ideas of difference. Many nursing behaviors were not simply due to a lack of cross-cultural knowledge. They were the product of staffing clinics in remote Aboriginal communities where change was difficult to accomplish and biomedical protocols took priority.

Most nurses who choose to work in remote communities started their career wanting to "make a difference" and improve the health of Aboriginal people. Upon their arrival in an Aboriginal community, many were convinced that small changes could lead to considerable progress. Altering the eating and hygiene habits of Aboriginal people, they believed, could drastically reduce morbidity and mortality. A young nurse reported that increased environmental health coupled with education and improved compliance would "make a real difference." What at first appeared to be simple changes, they quickly discovered, were difficult to accomplish. Damien (1998, 57) reports that nurses often feel upset because of an "inability to substantially change a situation that is not changeable." As a nurse's term progresses and community health fails to improve regardless of her efforts, she becomes more and more exasperated with Aboriginal people. Tina commented that when she first started nursing in the bush, she felt that substantial changes could be effected. As the years progressed, she realized that even a slight improvement in community-wide health outcomes would be tough to achieve. A problem that had at first seemed easy to solve quickly became insurmountable. Tina said, "After a while you realize you can't change things so you stop trying." Nurses wanted to improve health and when they were unable to do so because of the intractable nature of community lifestyles, they became frustrated. Brian commented, "This is why it is hard working out here. You do the best you can but they still die."

The everyday experiences of nurses and other non-Aboriginal staff shaped their responses and attitudes toward Aboriginal people, reinforcing differences between care providers and patients. Accepting generalizations regarding poor hygiene and health quickly leads to fatalism and therapeutic inertia (Hunter and Fagan 1994, 21). After casting Aboriginal people as resistant to change and improvement, it is a small step to form racial attitudes. While notions of race are grounded in wider Australian discourse about Aboriginal people, working in the clinic gave expression to these ideas. Frustration over the use of pharmaceuticals or after-hours callouts led to labels such as "chronically irresponsible" being applied indiscriminately to Aboriginal people.

Narratives of Aboriginal behaviors were marshaled by nursing staff to generate agency. In Lajamanu, conduct such as scolding patients was justified by invoking notions of Warlpiri inflexibility. Despite being informed of Warlpiri gender customs, some members of the non-Aboriginal medical staff chose to ignore these guidelines. Cultural awareness programs assume that once non-Aboriginal medical staff are made aware of local norms, they will be respected. In Lajamanu, this was not always the case. Disregarding Aboriginal beliefs was one way in which identity was publically demonstrated. Whiteness was performed through complaints of noncompliance, admonishing patients, and flouting Aboriginal social customs. Medical treatment became a venue through which race was enacted and ethnic identities were strengthened. Policies stressing the importance of cultural awareness fail to realize that the experience of providing medical care in the bush, coupled with essentialized notions of culture and the habitual performance of race, can constrain non-Aboriginal behaviors more than possessing knowledge of Aboriginal beliefs and norms.

Illness and Identity

Statistics highlighting the disparity between Aboriginal and non-Aboriginal health have been marshaled to argue for continuing legislative measures as well as increased funding, health education campaigns, and cross-cultural training. While health policies and medical interventions seek to improve rates of morbidity and mortality, they also help to shape and perpetuate notions of Aboriginality. In turn, these notions are manipulated and contested by Aboriginal people. Crandon-Malamud (1997, 86) writes, "Thus medicine plays a role in the formation (and reformation) of the meaning of ethnicity, and in effecting social change, particularly in an environment that is medically pluralistic and socially diverse." Surrounded by pervasive disparities, Aboriginal people use whatever tools are available as a means of reply, including illness. Consequently, struggles over identity can have a tremendous effect on health. To illustrate the way in which medical dialogues become the grounds for open conflict, I will examine concerns over, and responses to, poor child health.

Data indicates that Aboriginal child health is significantly behind that of the non-Aboriginal population. Indigenous children between the ages of one and fourteen are three times as likely to be treated for skin and parasitic diseases and twice as like to be treated for infectious disease (Pink and Allbon 2008, 92). In Aboriginal communities across Australia, a significant percentage of Aboriginal children "fail to thrive," not gaining weight and maturing as expected. Either lacking or not retaining the calories needed for growth, failure to thrive children have a greater risk for developmental and chronic disorders. In Alice Springs, 15 percent of children between the ages of one and five are malnourished (Russell et al. 2004, 187). For decades, health statistics and concerns over Aboriginal child health have inspired a number of government policies, including the decision in the early 1970s to allow Aboriginal Territorians to claim unemployment benefits without having been previously employed (Rowse 1998, 180). Today, improving child health remains a priority for the Northern Territory government (Northern Territory Department of Health 2005). While some interventions, such as the hospitalization of failure to thrive children, have proved an effective tool for increasing nutritional intake and growth, others have been less successful (Russell et al. 2004). The implementation and outcomes of child health initiatives provide a potent forum through which Aboriginal identity is constructed and maintained.

As part of the Northern Territory Emergency Response, the Lajamanu clinic began a healthy ear program designed to distribute oral antibiotics to children suffering from infections. When the healthy ear program was evaluated, Caroline reported that not a single child appeared to have been effectively treated. Despite the distribution of antibiotics, the children still suffered from infections. Nurses complained that the medication was not being administered properly by mothers. During the program, Caroline described how one mother violently threw the antibiotics in the rubbish bin before loudly exiting the clinic. Time after time, non-Aboriginal medical staff blamed the negligence of parents for poor child health, including failure to thrive. I was often told that Warlpiri people did not feed their children regularly or nutritiously. When working in the clinic, nurses made little or no effort to conceal their opinions. Caroline described a recent experience: While examining a small child, her colleague asked the mother how often the child was fed. The mother assured the nurse conducting the exam that the child was given food regularly. As soon as the exam was completed, the nurse turned to Caroline and said, "She says she fed her baby but clearly she didn't."

Nursing statements regarding child health illustrate the ways in which notions of ethnicity and race have been created and perpetuated via medical exchanges. Through interactions in the clinic, identity is enacted and "Aboriginal and non-Aboriginal people alike are called on to *navigate, inhabit and replenish* a complex set of signs as they represent themselves to each other" (Lea 2008, 157). Narratives of irresponsible mothers cast Aboriginal people as immoral, much in the same way that early twentieth century discussions of the "black pox" portrayed Aboriginal people as deviant. Nursing complaints regarding the health behavior of Aboriginal people continue to reflect earlier ideas that link Aboriginality, ill health, and a lack of "civilizing" values. Disparate rates of morbidity and mortality further naturalize ideas about a gap between Aboriginal and non-Aboriginal Australians. Medical statistics, policies, and interventions also persistently associate illness with Aboriginality. As a result, Aboriginal identity is stigmatized. By stigma, I am specifically referring to "bodily signs designed to expose something unusual and bad about the moral status of the signifier" (Goffman 1963, 11). In this sense, stigma is the product of enduring social relationships rather than isolated individual attributes. Already on the periphery, illness reinforces the social marginalization of Aboriginal people. For the residents of Lajamanu, disparities are experienced on a daily basis.

Racial difference is conspicuously present in the everyday life of Lajamanu. While the majority of the inhabitants were Aboriginal, all of the services—the store, the school, the clinic, the art center, the garage, and the outstation resource center—were managed by non-Aboriginal people. While Warlpiri people lived in overcrowded and poorly maintained homes, single non-Aboriginal workers resided in two-bedroom houses. While Aboriginal people received the majority of their income from government benefits, non-Aboriginal residents were steadily employed. While Warlpiri children attended the local school, non-Aboriginal residents, including teachers, chose to have their children attend the School of the Air, a radio-based education program located in Katherine. In addition to these visible disparities, a social apartheid seemed to be firmly entrenched. The inhabitants of Lajamanu rarely socialized across racial boundaries. I was told that for safety reasons, Aboriginal residents were not permitted to enter the nursing compound. During non-Aboriginal gatherings, participants would often sit behind a fence drinking beer while Warlpiri residents walked by, conscious of the heavy penalties Aboriginal people faced if they attempted to bring alcohol into the dry community. Everyday, Warlpiri people were plainly reminded that they endured living conditions, economic prospects, and educational opportunities that differed from those of non-Aboriginal Australians.

Surrounded by reminders of their status, Warlpiri people responded to the pervasive environment of social disparities. Lajamanu residents complained about government intervention, non-Aboriginal conduct, and persistent marginalization. Marshaling evidence of racial inequality, Aboriginal grievances were severe and relentless. The Intervention was a particularly inflammatory subject. While discussing his dislike for the policy of government-managed accounts, one man said, "They treat us like dogs because they think we are animals." Another man asserted, "They expect us to be *kardiya* straight out. No exceptions. It is genocide." Warlpiri reactions to illness were embedded within these larger narratives of white control and black subjugation. Themes of racial difference, inequality, and government management pervaded medical narratives. Non-Aboriginal medical staff were accused of racism, forcing treatment, experimenting on Aboriginal people, and disregarding the wishes of patients. In response, biomedical technologies and diagnoses could be cast as harmful. John stated that some pharmaceuticals were ineffective or toxic, while a *ngangkari* asserted that hospital medication had destroyed a portion of his healing power.

Portrayed as a reply to non-Aboriginal oppression and prejudice, Warlpiri people wielded health and illness as a tool of contestation by ignoring, critiquing, confronting, or repudiating the advice and behavior of medical staff. In so doing, Indigenous actions "seem to confirm the grotesque images of a deformed Aboriginality" (Cowlishaw 2004, 74). Persistently enacting a conventional discourse in which Aboriginal people are irresponsible, obscene, and incapable of "looking after" themselves, Lajamanu residents transformed their stigmatized identity into a source of power and resistance. By adopting illness as an identity and conforming to the stereotype of the noncompliant, chronically ill patient, Aboriginal people shocked and dismayed non-Aboriginal audiences, while garnering praise from Aboriginal ones. When Lily, a nurse, threatened Jeff, a diabetic, with the amputation of his foot if he did not begin to take his medication regularly, he replied that she could amputate the entire leg because he had no intention of being compliant. Lily could do little more than walk away dumbstruck. For several days, the story of Jeff's rebellion circulated among the Warlpiri population. Those recounting the tale often laughed as they stressed the stunned look that appeared on the Lily's face when she heard his reply. Far from being stigmatized for his behavior, Jeff was admired for his ability to displease the nurses.

Jeff's response to the threat of amputation was a potent demonstration of his identity as an Aboriginal man, a triumphant rejection of marginalization, and a forceful denial of vulnerability. However, this was not merely a struggle over meaning, confined to a war of words. Jeff's body and his life were at stake. As ill health, chronic disease, and noncompliance are transformed into indelible markers of Aboriginality, Warlpiri people have come to enact these traits in particular contexts. While shouting obscenities is one way in which the stigma of Aboriginality is performed and contested, illness is another. If being Aboriginal is synonymous with disease, embracing sickness can become a significant strategy. Throwing a child's medicine in the rubbish bin as non-Aboriginal medical staff watch is a powerful statement of Indigenous identity. Simultaneously affirming and rejecting physical and social suffering, Warlpiri people endure affliction.

Glossary

Warlpiri	English
jarnpa	Sorcerers
juju minyiminyi	Plant used to clear nasal congestion (biological name: *pterocaulon sphacelaturn*)
jukurrpa	Dreaming; a time during which ancestral beings roamed the landscape
kardiya	Individuals of European descent; white people
kardiya-kurlangu	Belonging to white people
kuku	Spirits of deceased individuals that roam around communities
kurruwalpa	Spirit being that implants *kuruwarri* into women to cause conception
kuruwarri	Customary law; designs; life force
kuyu	Meat and meat foodstuffs
milalpa	Spirits of ancestors which reside in, and protect, a kin group's country
minta	Bad cold or flu
miyi	Vegetable foods
ngangkari	Local healers capable of diagnosing and treating spiritual illness
ngarlu	Bush honey
nguwa	Healing power possessed by *ngangkari*
pama	Delicacy foods
pirlirrpa	Soul of living individuals
warnayarra	Rainbow serpent
yapa	Warlpiri, other Aboriginal, and Indigenous individuals
yapa-kurlangu	Belonging to *yapa*; Aboriginal way
yarda	Sharpened bone magically implanted to cause illness

Notes

CHAPTER 1

1. To protect privacy, all names are pseudonyms.
2. As proper adjectives describing a group of people, the words "Indigenous" and "Aboriginal" are capitalized.
3. There is no doubt that remote area clinics lack the resources of those in urban centers, but they are capable of treating most common ailments. While poor Indigenous health can be partially attributed to limited access to medical facilities and staff, I do not believe that this alone is capable of accounting for the significant difference in health disparities.
4. Yuendumu, a Warlpiri community in the southern Tanami, was established three years earlier. For additional details on the settlement of the region, see Chapter 2.
5. Consequently, most outstations and land claims are to the south of the community.
6. Warlpiri residents often asserted that there was not a single Aboriginal nurse or doctor in the Northern Territory.
7. Latz (1995, 62) has recorded over seventy plant species as being utilized for healing purposes, one-third of which can be found in the *Acacia* or *Eremophila* genus.
8. Heil and Macdonald (2008, 314) report similar responses in New South Wales.
9. As a non-Aboriginal anthropologist researching Aboriginal responses to illness, it was necessary to position myself within each of these groups. While I spent the majority of my time with Warlpiri people, it was also important that I maintain a social relationship with the non-Aboriginal nursing staff.
10. Gilligan (1997, 192) defines structural violence as "the increased rates of death and disability suffered by those who occupy the bottom rungs of society, as contrasted with the relatively lower death rates experienced by those who are above them."

CHAPTER 2

1. I believe George was referring to the work of Humphery, Dixon, and Marrawal (1998).

2. Despite the nutritional value of bush foods, dietary changes must be supplemented with increased exercise if morbidity is to be reduced (McDermott et al. 2000).

3. In Lajamanu, few residents live permanently on outstations. Those who do spend time at an outstation often prefer to move back and forth between the community and the bush.

4. Although the shop is technically owned by the community run Lajamanu Progress Association, grievances often stressed that the manager and senior staff were invariably non-Aboriginal.

5. Although accusations of price fixing have been recorded in other Aboriginal communities (Stewart 1997, 112), excessive price inflation seems doubtful as most stores show poor economic performance, producing only minimal profits (Young 1995, 231).

6. This expression is used not only in Lajamanu, but elsewhere in the Northern Territory. The origin of this phrase is obscure and there is no shortage of folk etymologies. On one occasion I was told that it simply referred to being low on money and food. On another occasion, I was informed that it was "Milo week," referring to the Nestlé® chocolate malt powder that is often mixed with milk or water: "We don't have any money so all we can have is Milo."

7. A survey of 3906 Aboriginal homes in the Northern Territory found that only 38 percent had facilities that would allow residents to prepare food effectively in the house, such as stoves, ovens, and water taps (Bailie and Runcie 2001, 366).

8. Obtaining transport to hunt and gather is a challenge for Aboriginal people throughout the Northern Territory (Beck 1985, 84; Povenelli 1993, 183; Tregenza and Abbot 1995, 19).

9. Similar constraints also affect the use of outstations.

CHAPTER 3

1. During the summer months, boys are initiated into manhood through sacred ceremonies in which the community participates.

2. The roles and abilities of Aboriginal healers have been examined anthropologically (Berndt and Berndt 1974; Cawte and Kidson 1964; Elkin 1994;

Gray 1979; Meggitt 1955; Spencer and Gillen 1904; Tonkinson 1978) and within the context of health care initiatives (Beck 1985; Devanesen 1985; Nathan and Leichleitner 1983; Taylor 1977; Tonkinson 1982).

3. Ethnographers have consistently reported that traditional Aboriginal healers lead a normal life without special privileges or status aside from their role in curing disease (Cawte and Kidson 1964, 977; Elkin 1994, 13; Mobbs 1991, 313; Tonkinson 1978, 107).

4. Meggitt (1955, 390) notes that each healer possesses several *maparnpa*, the substance that he says provides the ability to heal. In Warlpiri, *maparn* is a synonym of *ngangkari*, although the former is used far less frequently.

5. Cawte and Kidson (1964, 949) also record that *maparmpa* (healing power) is characterized by "animal qualities."

6. While both *ngangkari* and *jarnpa* are male, most people stated it was rare for one individual to possess *nguwa* and ensorcell others.

7. Over a hundred years ago, Spencer and Gillen (1904, 481) recounted the story of a man in Alice Springs losing his power as a result of drinking hot tea.

8. Top Springs Roadhouse and Katherine, approximately 300 and 600 kilometers distant, are the closest legal sources of alcohol.

9. Sorcerers have been described as part of the cosmologies of Aboriginal people living throughout the Central and Western Deserts including the Warlpiri (Cawte and Kidson 1964, 981; Meggitt 1955, 382-386), Kukatja (Peile 1997, 137), Mardudjara (Tonkinson 1978, 61), and Arrernte (Nathan and Leichleitner 1983, 78).

10. Elkin (1994, 50), Meggitt (1955, 387) and Tonkinson (1978, 111) note that beliefs regarding soul stealing were common in many parts of Australia.

11. Dreams commonly reveal the cause of sickness, particularly if sorcery is involved. Anthropologists have documented similar beliefs throughout the Western Desert (Dussart 2000; Elkin 1994, 40; Peile 1997, 116; Poirier 2005; Tonkinson 1982, 232).

12. Similarly, Schwarz (2010b, 67) notes that assertions of sorcery are increasing in Galiwin'ku where residents cited the rising rate of illness in the community and the high population density—thought to result in a higher number of interpersonal conflicts—as proof.

13. Throughout Central Australia, Aboriginal groups possess similar beliefs regarding ancestral spirits and ghosts (Cawte and Kidson 1964, 980; Meggitt 1955, 398; Nathan and Leichleitner 1983, 75; Peile 1997, 93; Tonkinson 1978, 86).

CHAPTER 4

1. The choice of treatment options based upon the diagnosis of spiritual or physical causes is described as occurring elsewhere in Australia (Gray 1979, 172; Nathan and Leichleitner 1983, 138; Tonkinson 1982, 239).

2. Gender issues surrounding clinical treatment of rural Aboriginal people are well documented (Bell 1982, 205; Devitt and McMasters 1998, 144; Eastwell 1973, 1015; Maher 1999, 232; Mobbs 1991, 317; Morgan, Slade, and Morgan 1997, 599; Nathan and Leichleitner 1983, 150; Tregenza and Abbot 1995, 26).

3. SLE patients in the United States, Canada, and the United Kingdom also used alternative medical therapies at higher rates than those without the disease (Moore et al. 2000).

4. It has been reported that patients have a tendency to consult the clinic immediately after being treated by a *ngangkari* in other regions of the Northern Territory as well (Cutter 1976, 38; Willis 1985, 28).

5. When an airplane is dispatched from Katherine to Lajamanu, it takes approximately an hour and a half to arrive. A nurse from Katherine accompanies every flight in the event that care is required en route. The rates of evacuation from Lajamanu vary from one every twenty days to over seven a week. Evacuations are provided free of charge to patients.

CHAPTER 5

1. Examining Navajo communities, Evaneshko (1993) notes that Native Americans tend to ignore or view as irrelevant many of the symptoms of diabetes.

2. Research has shown that noticeable symptoms were one of the main reasons Aboriginal people in the Northern Territory sought help in controlling diabetes (Scrimgeour, Rowse, and Lucas 1997, 48).

3. A lack of verbal confrontation does not indicate that either nurses or patients were satisfied with the experience or outcome of the consultation.

4. These attitudes are echoed by health advocates. Saggers and Gray (1991, 146) note that nurses can "have paternalistic if not racist attitudes."

CHAPTER 6

1. In 1953, mixed race individuals were given citizenship and allowed to work in hospitals. However, the majority of Aboriginal people in the Northern Territory did not benefit from this legislation (Kettle 1991, 2:290).

2. Basic skills included applying a simple dressing and sling; bandaging; taking a temperature and pulse; urine testing; hemoglobin estimations; controlling bleeding; resuscitation; treating animal bites, burns, fractures, eye injuries; identifying diarrhea, colds, STDs, urine infections, skin infections, malnutrition; administering injections; storing medicines; evacuating a patient; taking blood; possessing general nutrition information; and being able to drive, use a telephone, and a radio (Northern Territory Department of Health 1983).

3. Due to the social discomfort of working in a primarily female space with female supervisors, there is a higher turnover rate among male Aboriginal Health Workers throughout the Northern Territory (Tregenza and Abbot 1995, 20).

4. This issue seems to have persisted for over twenty years (Soong 1981, 186). Tregenza and Abbot (1995, 42) report that because most nurses assumed Aboriginal people would abuse usage privileges, possibly damaging the vehicle, nurses generally refused such requests, regardless of reason. Surveys show Aboriginal Health Workers feel this response is unfair (Josif and Elderton 1992, 55).

5. *Rdaka-rdaka wankami*, or literally "hands talking," is a comprehensive form of non-verbal expression, which is used most often when communicating over a long distance, hunting, during special ceremonial times, or mourning periods (Kendon 1988).

CHAPTER 7

1. Evaluators found that the program had not been put into action, little money had been allocated, local community involvement was non-existent, and it seemed that no one was accountable (Bhatia 1995, 8). The review made its own recommendations but these goals were also not implemented.

2. Examples include the *Aboriginal Health and Families: A Five Year Framework for Action* (Northern Territory Department of Health 2005) and *Closing the Gap between Indigenous and Non-Indigenous Australians* (Northern Territory Government 2007).

3. Environmental issues include: the supply of clean water and disposal of effluent and sewage; the control and dispersal of rubbish; the safe supply of electricity; the supply of cooking and heating fuel (wood); dog disease control; the maintenance of public health standards in public utilities (communal ablutions, stores, food outlets); dust control; reforestation and land management; the supply, maintenance, and repair of all health hardware

(e.g. functioning and hygienic bathrooms, laundries, toilets and kitchens); supply and maintenance of clean and dirty water; safe electrical fixtures; access to shade, wind and dust protection; house fencing; and household safety around the home and living area (Tregenza and Abbot 1995, 35).

4. This statistic includes participants in the Community Development Employment Program.

5. It is estimated that at least twenty serotypes of pneumococcus and fifty strains of non-typable *Haemophilus* are present in Aboriginal communities, far more than would be found in Darwin (Mathews 1996, 31).

6. In addition, individuals do not react uniformly to health messages or react in the way health professionals intend (Heil 2006, 106). Men's responses can differ from women's as can those of younger and older individuals.

References

Aboriginal and Torres Strait Islander Commission. 1994. *National Aboriginal and Torres Strait Islander Survey*. Canberra: Australian Bureau of Statistics.

Adams, V. 2002. "Establishing Proof: Translating 'Science' and the State in Tibetan Medicine." In *New Horizons in Medical Anthropology: Essays in Honor of Charles Leslie*, edited by C. M. Leslie, M. Nichter and M. Lock, 200–19. New York: Routledge.

Altman, Jon. 2003. "People on Country, Healthy Landscapes and Sustainable Indigenous Economic Futures: The Arnhem Land Case." *The Drawing Board: An Australian Review of Public Affairs* 4 (2): 65–82.

Anderson, Pat. 1996. "Priorities in Aboriginal Health." In *Aboriginal Health: Social and Cultural Transitions*, edited by G. Robinson, 15–18. Darwin: NTU Press.

Anderson, Warwick. 2006. *The Cultivation of Whiteness: Science, Health, and Racial Destiny in Australia*. Durham, NC: Duke University Press.

Arnold, David. 1993. *Colonizing the Body: State Medicine and Epidemic Disease in Nineteenth-Century India*. Berkeley: University of California Press.

Austin-Broos, Diane J. 1996a. "'Two Laws,' Ontologies, Histories: Ways of Being Arrernte Today." *The Australian Journal of Anthropology* 7:1–20.

———. 1996b. "What's in a Time or Place? Reflections on Swain's Hypothesis." *Social Analysis* 40:3–9.

———. 2009. *Arrernte Present, Arrernte Past: Invasion, Violence, and Imagination in Indigenous Central Australia*. Chicago: University of Chicago Press.

Australian Bureau of Statistics. 2002. *National Aboriginal and Torres Strait Island Social Survey, Northern Territory*. Canberra: Australian Bureau of Statistics.

———. 2006. *National Aboriginal and Torres Strait Islander Health Survey 2004–05, Northern Territory*. Canberra: Australian Bureau of Statistics.

———. 2009. *Experimental Life Tables for Aboriginal and Torres Strait Islander Australians, 2005–2007*. Canberra: Australian Bureau of Statistics.

Australian Medical Association. 2002. *Public Report Card 2002: Aboriginal and Torres Strait Islander Health—No More Excuses*. Canberra: Australian Medical Association.

Bailie, Ross, and Myfanwy Runcie. 2001. "Household Infrastructure in Aboriginal Communities and the Implications for Health Improvement." *Medical Journal of Australia* 175 (7): 363–6.

Bailie, Ross, and Kayli J. Wayte. 2006. "Housing and Health in Indigenous Communities: Key Issues for Housing and Health Improvement in Remote Aboriginal and Torres Strait Islander Communities." *Australian Journal of Rural Health* 14:178–83.

Bartlett, Ben. 1996. "Aboriginal Community Control: Is It Just Rhetoric?" In *Aboriginal Health: Social and Cultural Transitions*, edited by G. Robinson, 207–13. Darwin: Northern Territory University Press.

Bartlett, Ben, and David Legge. 1994. *Beyond the Maze: Proposals for a More Effective Administration of Aboriginal Health Programs.* Canberra: Australian National University.

Bashford, Alison. 2000. "'Is White Australia Possible?' Race, Colonialism and Tropical Medicine." *Ethnic and Racial Studies* 23 (2): 248–71.

Batchelor College. 1995. *School of Health Studies, Batchelor College.* Batchelor, N.T.: Batchelor College.

Beck, Eduard. 1985. *The Enigma of Aboriginal Health: Interaction between Biological, Social and Economic Factors in Alice Springs Town-Camps.* Canberra: Australian Institute of Aboriginal Studies.

Beckett, Jeremy. 1993. "Walter Newton's History of the World—or Australia." *American Ethnologist* 20 (4): 675–95.

———. 2010. "National Anthropologies and Their Problems." In *Culture Crisis: Anthropology and Politics in Aboriginal Australia*, edited by J. Altman and M. Hinkson, 32–45. Sydney: University of New South Wales.

Bell, Diane. 1982. "Women's Changing Role in Health Maintenance in a Central Australian Community." In *Body, Land and Spirit: Health and Healing in Aboriginal Society*, edited by J. Reid. St. Lucia: University of Queensland Press.

Berndt, Catherine. 1964. "The Role of Native Doctors in Aboriginal Australia." In *Magic, Faith and Healing: Studies in Primitive Psychiatry Today*, edited by A. Kiev. New York: The Free Press.

Berndt, Ronald M. 1974. "Wuradjeri Magic and 'Clever Men.'" *Oceania* 18 (1): 4–17.

Berndt, Ronald, and Catherine Berndt. 1974. *The First Australians.* Sydney: Ure Smith.

Bhatia, Kuldeep. 1995. "National Aboriginal Health Strategy Evaluation 1994." *Aboriginal and Torres Strait Islander Health Information Bulletin* 21:4–10.

Bibeau, G., and D. Pedersen. 2002. "A Return to Scientific Racism in Medical Social Sciences: The Case of Sexuality and the AIDS Epidemic in Africa." In *New Horizons in Medical Anthropology: Essays in Honor of Charles Leslie*, edited by M. Nichter and M. Lock, 141–71. New York: Routledge.

Bird, Douglas, Rebecca Bleige Bird, and Christopher H. Parker. 2005. "Aboriginal Burning Regimes and Hunting Strategies in Australia's Western Desert." *Human Ecology* 33 (4): 443–64."

Board of Inquiry into the Protection of Aboriginal Children from Sexual Abuse. 2007. *Ampe Akelyernemane Meke Mekarle "Little Children Are Sacred."* Darwin: Northern Territory Government.

Brady, Maggie, Stephen Kunitz, and David Nash. 1997. "WHO's Definition?: Australian Aborigines, Conceptualisations of Health and the World Health Organization." In *Migrants, Minorities and Health: Historical and Contemporary Studies*, edited by L. Marks and M. Worboys, 272–90. London: Routledge.

Briggs, Charles, and Clara Mantini-Briggs. 2003. *Stories in the Time of Cholera: Racial Profiling During a Medical Nightmare.* Berkeley: University of California Press.

Brimblecombe, Julie K., and Kerin O'Dea. 2009. "The Role of Energy Cost in Food Choices for an Aboriginal Population in Northern Australia." *Medical Journal of Australia* 190:549–51.

Buchler, I., and K. Maddock, eds. 1978. *The Rainbow Serpent: A Chromatic Piece.* The Hague: Mouton.

Burnett, Rod. 1996. "Both Ways." *Aboriginal and Islander Health Worker Journal* 20 (2): 9.

Butler, Judith. 1997. *Excitable Speech: A Politics of the Performative.* New York: Routledge.

Caldwell, John C., Pat Caldwell, and Pat Quiggin. 1989. "The Social Context of AIDS in Sub-Saharan Africa." *Population and Development Review* 15 (2): 185–234.

Carnegie, David. 1898. *Spinifex and Sand.* London: C. Arthur Pearson.

Carpenter-Song, Elizabeth A., Megan Nordquest Schwallie, and Jeffrey Longhofer. 2007. "Cultural Competence Reexamined: Critique and Directions for the Future." *Psychiatric Services* 58 (10): 1362–5.

Cawte, John. 1965. "Medicine Man, Medical Man." *Medical Journal of Australia* 2 (3): 134–6.

———. 1974. *Medicine is the Law: Studies in the Psychiatric Anthropology of Australian Tribal Societies.* Adelaide: Rigby Press.

Cawte, John, and M. A. Kidson. 1964. "Australian Ethnopsychiatry: The Warlpiri Doctor." *Medical Journal of Australia* 2 (25): 977–83.

Christen, Kimberley. 2009. *Aboriginal Business: Alliances in a Remote Australian Town.* Santa Fe, NM: School for Advanced Research Press.

Clements, Forrest E. 1932. *Primitive Concepts of Disease.* Berkeley: University of California Press.

Collins, Emma, and Mark Warcon. 1994. "Aboriginal Studies and Environmental Health." *Aboriginal and Islander Health Worker Journal* 18 (1): 7–8.

Collmann, Jeff. 1988. *Fringe-Dwellers and Welfare: The Aboriginal Response to Bureaucracy.* St. Lucia: University of Queensland Press.

Comaroff, Jean. 1993. "The Diseased Heart of Africa: Medicine, Colonialism and the Black Body." In *Knowledge, Power, and Practice: The Anthropology of Medicine and Everyday Life*, edited by S. Lindenbaum and M. Lock, 305–29. Berkeley: University of California Press.

Comaroff, Jean, and John Comaroff. 1991. *Of Revelation and Revolution, Volume 1: Christianity, Colonialism, and Consciousness in South Africa*. Chicago: University of Chicago Press.

Comaroff, John, and Jean Comaroff. 1992. *Ethnography and the Historical Imagination*. Boulder, CO: Westview Press.

Correy, Simon. 2006. "The Reconstruction of Aboriginal Sociality through the Identification of Traditional Owners in New South Wales." *The Australian Journal of Anthropology* 17 (3): 336–47.

Cowlishaw, Gillian. 1986. "Aborigines and Anthropologists." *Australian Aboriginal Studies* 1:2–12.

———. 2001. "Race at Work: Reflecting on Fieldwork in the Northern Territory." *Journal of the Royal Anthropological Institute (N.S.)* 3:95–113.

———. 2004. *Blackfellas, Whitefellas, and the Hidden Injuries of Race*. Oxford: Blackwell Publishing.

———. 2010. "Helping Anthropologists, Still." In *Culture Crisis: Anthropology and Politics in Aboriginal Australia*, edited by J. Altman and M. Hinkson, 46–60. Sydney: University of New South Wales.

Cramer, Jennifer. 1995. "Finding Solutions to Support Remote Area Nurses." *Australian Nursing Journal* 2 (6): 21–25.

———. 2005. *Sounding the Alarm: Remote Area Nurses and Aboriginals at Risk*. Crawley, W.A.: University of Western Australia Press.

Crandon-Malamud, Libbet. 1993. *From the Fat of Our Souls: Social Change, Political Process and Medical Pluralism in Bolivia*. Berkeley: University of California Press.

———. 1997. "Phantoms and Physicians: Social Change through Medical Pluralism." In *The Anthropology of Medicine: From Culture to Method*, edited by L. Romanucci-Ross, D. Moerman and L. Tancredi, 85–112. New York: Bergin & Garvey.

Csordas, Thomas. 1990. "Embodiment as a Paradigm for Anthropology." *Ethos* 18 (1): 5–47.

Curtin Indigenous Research Centre. 2000. *Training Re-Visions: A National Review of Aboriginal and Torres Strait Islander Health Worker Training*. Canberra: Office for Aboriginal and Torres Strait Islander Health.

Cutter, Trevor. 1976. *Report on Community Health Model: Health by the People of the Central Australian Aboriginal Congress*. Alice Springs: Central Australian Aboriginal Congress.

d'Abbs, Peter. 1998. *Revised Local Evaluation Plan for the Katherine West Region Coordinated Care Trial*. Darwin: Menzies School of Health Research.

d'Abbs, Peter, Samantha Tongi, Joseph Fitz, Ross Bailie, Suzie Adsett, Letitia Del Fabbro, Noni Wales, and John Deeble. 2000. *Jirntangku Miyrta Katherine West Coordinated Care Trial Local Evaluation Final Report.* Darwin: Menzies School of Health Research.

DaCosta, Cheryl. 1996. "Promoting Health Both Ways." *Aboriginal and Islander Health Worker Journal* 20 (2): 14–15.

Damien, Howard. 1998. *More than Just a Nurse: A Support Manual for Remote Area Nurses Working in Aboriginal Communities of the Top End of the NT.* Darwin: Territory Health Services.

Department of Health/Department of Aboriginal Affairs. Joint Ministerial Evaluation Team. 1982. *Report on Three Rural Community Controlled Aboriginal Health Services in Central Australia 1978–1981.* Canberra: Department of Health.

Desjarlais, Robert. 1996. "Struggling Along." In *Things as They Are: New Directions in Phenomenological Anthropology*, edited by M. Jackson, 70–93. Bloomington: Indiana University Press.

———. 1997. *Shelter Blues: Sanity and Selfhood among the Homeless.* Philadelphia: University of Pennsylvania Press.

Devanesen, Dayalan. 1982. "The Aboriginal Health Worker Training Programme in Central Australia." *Panacea* 13 (1): 14–22.

———. 1985. "Traditional Aboriginal Medicine and Bi-Cultural Approaches to Health Care in Australia's Northern Territory." In *Alcohol and Drug Use in a Changing Society*, edited by K. P. Larkins, D. McDonald, and C. Watson, 33–41. Canberra: National Drug Institute.

Devanesen, Dayalan, and Patrick Maher. 2003. "Traditional Aboriginal Health Practice in Australia." In *Medicine across Cultures: History and Practice of Medicine in Non-Western Cultures*, edited by Helaine Selin, 175–90. New York: Springer Press.

Devitt, Jeannie, and Anthony McMasters. 1998. *Living on Medicine: A Cultural Study of End-Stage Renal Disease among Aboriginal People.* Alice Springs: IAD Press.

Durie, Mason. 2009. "Maori Health 2035." Paper read at Te ORA 'Whiti ki te Ao Marama'—'Determining Our Future,' at Wellington, New Zealand.

Dussart, Francoise. 2000. *The Politics of Ritual in an Aboriginal Settlement: Kinship, Gender and the Currency of Knowledge.* Washington DC: Smithsonian Institution Press.

———. 2009. "Diet, Diabetes, and Relatedness in a Central Australian Aboriginal Settlement: Some Qualitative Recommendations to Facilitate the Creation of Culturally-Sensitive Health Promotion Initiatives." *Health Promotion Journal of Australia* 20 (3): 202–7.

———. 2010. "'It is Hard to Be Sick Now': Diabetes and The Reconstruction of Indigenous Sociality." *Anthropologica* 52 (1): 77–85.

Eastwell, Harry D. 1973. "The Traditional Healer in Modern Arnhem Land." *Medical Journal of Australia* 2:1011–7.

Elkin, A. P. 1994. *Aboriginal Men of High Degree*. St. Lucia: University of Queensland Press.

Esterman, Adrian, and David Ben-Tovim. 2002. "The Australian Coordinated Care Trials: Success or Failure?" *Medical Journal of Australia* 177 (9): 469–70.

Evaneshko, Veronica. 1993. "Presenting Complaints in a Navajo Indian Diabetic Population." In *Diabetes as a Disease Of Civilization: The Impact of Culture Change on Indigenous Peoples*, edited by J. R. Joe and R. S. Young, 357–77. New York: Walter de Gruyter and Co.

Farley, John. 1991. *Bilharzia: A History of Imperial Tropical Medicine*. Cambridge: Cambridge University Press.

Farmer, Paul. 1999. *Infections and Inequalities: The Modern Plagues*. Berkeley: University of California Press.

———. 2003. *Pathologies of Power: Health, Human Rights, and the New War on the Poor*. Berkeley: University of California Press.

Fassin, Didier. 2007. *When Bodies Remember: Experiences and Politics of AIDS in South Africa*. Berkeley: University of California Press.

Ferguson, James. 1990. *The Anti-Politics Machine: "Development," Depoliticization and Bureaucratic State Power in Lesotho*. Cambridge: Cambridge University Press.

Ferreira, Mariana Leal, and Gretchen Chesley Lang. 2006. "Introduction: Deconstructing Diabetes." In *Indigenous People and Diabetes: Community Empowerment and Wellness*, edited by M. L. Ferreira and G. C. Lang, 3–20. Durham, NC: Carolina Academic Press.

Figlio, Karl. 1976. "The Metaphor of Organization: An Historiographical Perspective on the Bio-Medical Sciences of the Early Nineteenth Century." *History of Science* 14:17–53.

Flick, Barbara. 1997. "'Empowering' Aboriginal Health Workers: As Victims—or Controllers of Our Destiny?" *Aboriginal and Islander Health Worker Journal* 21 (3): 19–21.

Flick, Barbara, and Brendan Nelson. 1994. "Land and Indigenous Health." *Land, Rights, Laws* 3:1–8.

Food and Nutrition Unit. 1998. *Survey of Northern Territory Remote Community Stores*. Darwin: Territory Health Services.

Foucault, Michel. 1973. *The Birth of the Clinic: An Archaeology of Medical Perception*. Translated by A. M. Sheridan Smith. London: Tavistock.

Garro, Linda. 2000. "Cultural Knowledge as Resource in Illness Narratives." In *Narrative and the Cultural Construction of Illness and Healing*, edited by C. Mattingly and L. Garro, 70–87. Berkeley: University of California Press.

Garro, Linda, and Gretchen Chesley Lang. 1993. "Explanations of Diabetes: Anishinaabeg and Dakota Deliberate upon a New Illness." In *Diabetes as a Disease of Civilization: The Impact of Culture Change on Indigenous Peoples*, edited by J. R. Joe and R. S. Young, 293–328. New York: Walter de Gruyter and Co.

Geest, Sjaak van der. 2005. "'Sacraments' in the Hospital: Exploring the Magic and Religion of Recovery." *Anthropology & Medicine* 12 (2): 135–50.

Geest, Sjaak van der, and Susan Reynolds Whyte. 1989. "The Charm of Medicines: Metaphors and Metonyms." *Medical Anthropology Quarterly* 3 (4): 345–67.

Giles, E. 1889. *Australia Twice Traversed*. London: Sampson, Low, Marston and Rivington.

Gillespie, James. 1991. *The Price of Health: Australian Governments and Medical Politics 1910–1960*. Cambridge: Cambridge University Press.

Gilligan, James. 1997. *Violence: Reflections on a National Epidemic*. New York: Vintage.

Gluckman, Max. 1940. "Analysis of a Social Situation in Modern Zululand." *Bantu Studies* 14:1–30, 147–74.

Goffman, Erving. 1963. *Stigma: Notes on the Management of Spoiled Identity*. New York: Simon & Schuster.

Good, Byron. 1994. *Medicine, Rationality and Experience: An Anthropological Perspective*. Cambridge: Cambridge University Press.

Gordon, Deborah. 1988. "Tenacious Assumptions in Western Medicine." In *Biomedicine Examined*, edited by M. Lock and D. Gordon, 19–56. Dordrecht: Kluwer Academic Publishers.

Gordon, Elisa. 2000. "Preventing Waste: A Ritual Analysis of Candidate Selection for Kidney Transplantation. *Anthropology & Medicine* 7 (3): 351–72.

Graham, M. 2002. "Food, Health, and Identity in a Rural Andean Community." In *Medical Pluralism in the Andes*, edited by J. D. Koss-Chioino, T. Leatherman and C. Greenway, 148–65. New York: Routledge.

Gray, Dennis. 1979. "Traditional Medicine on the Carnarvon Aboriginal Reserve." In *Aborigines of the West*, edited by R. Berndt, 169–83. Nedlands: University of Western Australia Press.

Grootjans, John, and Michele Spiers. 1996. "'Both Ways' in Aboriginal and Torres Strait Islander Health Worker Education." *Aboriginal and Islander Health Worker Journal* 20 (4): 11–13.

Hamrosi, K., S. J. Taylor, and P. Aslani. 2006. "Issues with Prescribed Medications in Aboriginal Communities: Aboriginal Health Workers' Perspectives." *Rural and Remote Health* 6:557–70.

Harloe, Lorraine. 1991. "Anton Breinl and the Australian Institute of Tropical Medicine." In *Health and Healing in Tropical Australia and Papua New Guinea*, edited by R. Macleod and D. Denoon, 35–46. Townsville, QLD: James Cook University Press.

Harrington, Zinta, David P. Thomas, Bart J. Currie, and Joy Bulkanhawuy. 2006. "Challenging Perceptions of Non-Compliance with Rheumatic Fever Prophylaxis in a Remote Aboriginal Community." *Medical Journal of Australia* 184 (10): 514–7.

Harrison, Lindsey. 1991. "Food, Nutrition and Growth in Aboriginal Communities." In *The Health of Aboriginal Australia*, edited by J. Reid, 123–72. Marrickville, N.S.W.: Harcourt Brace Jovanovich.

Health Professions Licensing Authority. 2008. *Aboriginal Health Worker Code of Ethics*. Northern Territory Government. *www.health.nt.gov.au/library/scripts/ objectifyMedia.aspx?file=pdf/12/50.pdf&siteID=1&str_title=AHW Code Of Ethics.pdf*.

———. 2010. *Aboriginal Health Worker Register as at March 2010*. Northern Territory Government *www.health.nt.gov.au/library/scripts/objectifyMedia. aspx?file=pdf/32/15.pdf&siteID=1&str_title=AHW Register.pdf*. Accessed October 1, 2010.

Heil, Daniela. 2006. "Shifting Expectations of Treatment: From 'Patient as Individual' to 'Patient as Social Person.'" *Australian Aboriginal Studies* 2006 (2): 98–110.

———. 2009. "Embodied Selves and Social Selves: Aboriginal Well-Being in Rural New South Wales, Australia." In *Pursuits of Happiness: Well-Being in Anthropological Perspective*, edited by G. Mathews and C. Izquierdo, 88–108. New York: Berghahn Books.

Heil, Daniela, and Gaynor Macdonald. 2008. "'Tomorrow Comes When Tomorrow Comes': Managing Aboriginal Health within an Ontology of Life-as-Contingent." *Oceania* 78:299–319.

Hinkson, Melinda. 2010. "Introduction: Anthropology and the Culture Wars." In *Culture Crisis: Anthropology and Politics in Aboriginal Australia*, edited by J. Altman and M. Hinkson, 1–17. Sydney: University of New South Wales Press.

Hoy, Wendy E., Srinivas Kondalsamy-Chennakesavan, Zhiqiang Wang, Esther Briganti, Jonathan Shaw, Kevan Polkinghorne, and Steven Chadban. 2007. "Quantifying the Excess Risk for Proteinuria, Hypertension and Diabetes in Australian Aborigines: Comparison of Profiles in Three Remote Communities in the Northern Territory with Those in the AusDiab Study." *Australian and New Zealand Journal of Public Health* 31 (2): 177–83.

Hughes, Helen. 2007. *Lands of Shame: Aboriginal and Torres Strait Islander "Homelands" in Transition*. Sydney: Federation Press.

Humphery, Kim. 2001. "Dirty Questions: Indigenous Health and 'Western Research.'" *Australia and New Zealand Journal of Public Health* 25 (3): 197–202.

————. 2006. "Culture Blindness? Aboriginal Health, 'Patient Non-Compliance' and the Conceptualisation of Difference in Australia's Northern Territory." In *Indigenous People and Diabetes: Community Empowerment and Wellness*, edited by M. L. Ferreira and G. C. Lang, 493–509. Durham, NC: Carolina Academic Press.

Humphery, Kim, Mervyn Dixon, and James Marrawal. 1998. *From the Bush to the Store: Diabetes, Everyday Life and the Critique of Health Services in Two Remote Northern Territory Aboriginal Communities*. Darwin: Diabetes Research Trust.

Hunter, Ernest. 1993. *Aboriginal Health and History: Power and Prejudice in Remote Australia*. Cambridge: Cambridge University Press.

Hunter, Ernest, and Patricia Fagan. 1994. "White Dreaming: Stereotypes of Aboriginal People in Medical Practice." *Aboriginal and Torres Strait Islander Health Information Bulletin* 19:17–24.

Jackson, M. Yvonne. 1993. "Diet, Culture, and Diabetes." In *Diabetes as a Disease of Civilization: The Impact of Culture Change on Indigenous Peoples*, edited by J. R. Joe and R. S. Young, 381–406. New York: Walter de Gruyter and Co.

Jackson, Michael. 1989. *Paths toward a Clearing: Radical Empiricism and Ethnographical Inquiry*. Bloomington: Indiana University Press.

————. 1996. "Phenomenology, Radical Empiricism, and Anthropological Critique." In *Things as They Are: New Directions in Phenomenological Anthropology*, edited by M. Jackson, 1–50. Bloomington: Indiana University Press.

Janzen, John M. 1978. "The Comparative Study of Medical Systems as Changing Social Systems." *Social Science and Medicine* 12 (2B): 121–9.

Jay, S., I. F. Litt, and R. H. Durant. 1984. "Compliance with Therapeutic Regimes." *Journal of Adolescent Health Care* 5 (2): 124–36.

Jebb, Mary Anne. 2002. *Blood, Sweat and Welfare: A History of White Bosses and Aboriginal Pastoral Workers*. Nedlands, W.A.: University of Western Australia Press.

Jenks, Angela C. 2011. "From 'Lists of Traits' to 'Open-Mindedness': Emerging Issues in Cultural Competence Education." *Culture, Medicine and Psychiatry* 35:209–35.

Jochelson, Karen. 2001. *The Colour of Disease: Syphilis and Racism in South Africa, 1880–1950*. New York: Palgrave.

Josif, Paul, and Cath Elderton. 1992. *Working Together? A Review of Aboriginal Health Workers in Australia's Top End*. Darwin: Department of Health and Community Services.

Kaberry, Phyllis. 1939. *Aboriginal Women, Sacred and Profane*. London: Routledge.

Katherine West Health Board. 2003. *Something Special: The Inside Story of the Katherine West Health Board*. Canberra: Aboriginal Studies Press.

Kendon, Adam. 1988. *Sign Languages of Aboriginal Australia: Cultural, Semiotic and Communicative Perspectives*. Cambridge: Cambridge University Press.

Kennedy, Kate. 1997. *Quality Discharge Planning: Doing It Better for the Bush*. Darwin: Territory Health Services.

Kettle, Ellen. 1991. *Health Services in the Northern Territory: A History 1824–1970. Vol. 1*. Darwin: Australian National University Press.

———. 1991. *Health Services in the Northern Territory: A History 1824–1970. Vol. 2*. Darwin: Australian National University Press.

Kleinman, Arthur, and Peter Benson. 2006a. "Anthropology in the Clinic: The Problem of Cultural Competency and How to Fix It." *PLoS Medicine* 3 (10): 1673–6.

———. 2006b. "Culture, Moral Experience and Medicine." *The Mount Sinai Journal of Medicine* 73 (6): 834–9.

Kleinman, Arthur, and Joan Kleinman. 1996. "Suffering and Its Professional Transformation: Toward an Ethnography of Interpersonal Experience." In *Things as They Are: New Directions in Phenomenological Anthropology*, edited by M. Jackson, 169–95. Bloomington: Indiana University Press.

Kowal, Emma. 2010. "Is Culture the Problem or the Solution? Outstation Health and the Politics of Remoteness." In *Culture Crisis: Anthropology and Politics in Aboriginal Australia*, edited by J. Altman and M. Hinkson, 179–94. Sydney: University of New South Wales.

Kowal, Emma, and Yin Paradies. 2010. "Enduring Dilemmas of Indigenous Health." *Medical Journal of Australia* 192 (10): 599–600.

Kruske, S. G., A. R. Ruben, and D. R. Brewster. 1999. "An Iron Treatment Trial in an Aboriginal Community: Improving Non-Adherence." *Journal of Paediatrics and Child Health* 35:153–8.

Kuper, Adam. 1999. *Culture: The Anthropologists' Account*. Cambridge, MA: Harvard University Press.

Lang, Gretchen Chesley. 2006. "Talking about a New Illness with the Dakota: Reflections on Diabetes, Foods, and Culture." In *Indigenous People and Diabetes: Community Empowerment and Wellness*, edited by M. L. Ferreira and G. C. Lang, 203–31. Durham, NC: Carolina Academic Press.

Langford, Jean M. 2002. *Fluent Bodies: Ayurvedic Remedies for Postcolonial Imbalance*. Durham, NC: Duke University Press.

Lattas, Andrew, and Barry Morris. 2010. "The Politics of Suffering and the Politics of Anthropology." In *Culture Crisis: Anthropology and Politics in Aboriginal Australia*, edited by J. Altman and M. Hinkson, 61–87. Sydney: University of New South Wales Press.

Latz, Peter. 1995. *Bushfires and Bushtucker: Aboriginal Plant Use in Central Australia*. Alice Springs: IAD Press.

Lea, Tess. 2008. *Bureaucrats and Bleeding Hearts: Indigenous Health in Northern Australia*. Sydney: University of New South Wales Press.

Lea, Tess, and Paul Pholeros. 2010. "This is Not a Pipe: The Treacheries of Indigenous Housing." *Public Culture* 22 (1): 187–211.

Lee, Amanda J., Dympna Leonard, Aletia A. Moloney, and Deanne L. Minniecon. 2009. "Improving Aboriginal and Torres Strait Islander Nutrition and Health." *Medical Journal of Australia* 190 (10): 547–8.

Lee, Gina, and David Morris. 2005. *Best Practice Models for Effective Consultation: Towards Improving Built Environment Outcomes for Remote Indigenous Communities*. Melbourne: Australian Housing and Urban Research Institute.

Lewis, Gilbert. 1993. "Double Standards of Treatment Evaluation." In *Knowledge, Power and Practice: The Anthropology of Medicine of Everyday Life*, edited by S. Lindenbaum and M. Lock, 189–218. Berkeley: University of California Press.

Macklin, Jenny. 2008. *Budget: Closing the Gap between Indigenous and Non-Indigenous Australians*. Barton ACT: Commonwealth of Australia.

Macleod, Catriona, and Kevin Durrheim. 2002. "Racializing Teenage Pregnancy: 'Culture' and 'Tradition' in the South Africa Scientific Literature." *Ethnic and Racial Studies* 25 (5): 778–801.

Maher, Patrick. 1999. "A Review of 'Traditional' Aboriginal Health Beliefs." *Australian Journal of Rural Health* 7:229–36.

Malik, Kenan. 1996. *The Meaning of Race: Race, History, and Culture in Western Society*. Houndmills, Basingstoke: Macmillan.

Marshall, Wende Elizabeth. 2005. "AIDS, Race and the Limits of Science." *Social Science and Medicine* 60:2515–25.

Mathews, John. 1996. "Aboriginal Health: Historical, Social and Cultural Influences. In *Aboriginal Health: Social and Cultural Transitions*, edited by G. Robinson, 29–38. Darwin: Northern Territory University Press.

May, D. 1994. *Aboriginal Labour and the Cattle Industry: Queensland from White Settlement to the Present*. Cambridge: Cambridge University Press.

McDermott, Robyn, Kevin Rowley, Amanda Lee, Sabina Knight, and Kerin O'Dea. 2000. "Increase in Prevalence of Obesity and Diabetes and Decrease in Plasma Cholesterol in a Central Australian Aboriginal Community." *Medical Journal of Australia* 172 (10): 480–4.

McDonald, Heather. 2001. *Blood, Bones, and Spirit: Aboriginal Christianity in an East Kimberley Town*. Melbourne: Melbourne University Press.

———. 2010. "Universalising the Particular? God and Indigenous Spirit Beings in East Kimberley." *The Australian Journal of Anthropology* 21:51–70.

McGregor, Russell. 1997. *Imagined Destinies: Aboriginal Australians and the Doomed Race Theory, 1880–1939*. Carlton, Vic.: Melbourne University Press.

Meggitt, Mervyn. 1955. "Djanba among the Walbiri, Central Australia." *Anthropos* 50 (3):375–403.

———. 1962. *Desert People: A Study of the Walbiri Aborigines of Central Australia*. Sydney: Angus and Robertson.

Merlan, Francesca. 1986. "Australian Aboriginal Conception Beliefs Revisited." *Man* 21 (3): 474–93.

———. 2000. "Representing the Rainbow: Aboriginal Culture in an Interconnected World. *Australian Aboriginal Studies* 1 & 2:20–6.

———. 2005. "Explorations towards Intercultural Accounts of Socio-Cultural Reproduction and Change." *Oceania* 75 (3): 167–82.

Mitchell, Jessie. 2007. "History." In *Social Determinants of Indigenous Health*, edited by B. Carson, 41–64. Crows Nest, N.S.W.: Allen & Unwin.

Mobbs, Robyn. 1991. "In Sickness and in Health: The Sociocultural Context of Aboriginal Well-Being, Illness and Healing." In *The Health of Aboriginal Australia*, edited by J. Reid, 292–325. Marrickville, N.S.W.: Harcourt Brace Jovanovich.

Montagu, Ashley. 1974. *Coming into Being among the Australian Aborigines: A Study of Procreative Beliefs of the Native Tribes of Australia*. London: Routledge and Kegan Paul.

Moore, Andrew, Michelle Petri, Susan Manzi, David Isenberg, Caroline Gordon, and Jean-Luc Senecal. 2000. "The Use of Alternative Medical Therapies in Patients with Systematic Lupus Erythematosus." *Arthritis & Rheumatism* 43 (6): 1410–8.

Morgan, Douglas, Malcolm Slade, and Catherine Morgan. 1997. "Aboriginal Philosophy and Its Impact on Health Care Outcomes." *Australian and New Zealand Journal of Public Health* 21 (6): 597–601.

Morgan, George. 2006. *Unsettled Places: Aboriginal People and Urbanisation in New South Wales*. Kent Town, S.A.: Wakefield.

Munn, Nancy. 1973. *Walbiri Iconography: Graphic Representation and Cultural Symbolism in a Central Australian Society*. Ithaca, NY: Cornell University Press.

Musharbash, Yasmine. 2004. "Red Bucket for the Red Cordial, Green Bucket for the Green Cordial: On the Logic and Logistics of Warlpiri Birthday Parties." *Australian Journal of Anthropology* 15:12–22.

———. 2009. *Yuendumu Everyday: Contemporary Life in Remote Aboriginal Australia*. Canberra: Aboriginal Studies Press.

Myers, Fred. 1985. "Illusion and Reality: Aboriginal Self-Determination in Central Australia." In *The Future of Former Foragers in Australia and Southern Africa*, edited by C. Schrire and R. Gordon, 109–22. Cambridge, MA: Cultural Survival.

————. 1986. *Pintupi Country, Pintupi Self: Sentiment, Place, and Politics among Western Desert Aborigines*. Washington DC: Smithsonian Institution Press.

Nathan, Pam, and Dick Leichleitner. 1983. *Health Business*. Richmond, Vic: Heinemann Educational Australia.

National Aboriginal Community Controlled Health Organisation. 2007. *National Aboriginal Community Controlled Health Organisation Achievements: Aboriginal People Making the Health System Equitable*. Sydney: National Aboriginal Community Controlled Health Organisation.

National Aboriginal Health Strategy Evaluation Committee. 1994. *The National Aboriginal Health Strategy: An Evaluation*. Canberra: Commonwealth of Australia.

National Aboriginal Health Strategy Working Party. 1989. *The National Aboriginal Health Strategy*. Canberra: Commonwealth of Australia.

Naughton, Joan, Kerin O'Dea, and Andrew Sinclair. 1986. "Animal Foods in Traditional Aboriginal Diets: Polyunsaturated and Low in Fat." *Lipids* 21: 684–90.

Northern Territory Aboriginal Health Worker Conference. 1988. "Northern Territory Aboriginal Health Worker Conference Report, Tuesday 23 August 1988 to Thursday 25 August 1998." Paper read at Northern Territory Aboriginal Health Worker Conference, at Darwin, Australia.

Northern Territory Department of Health. 1983. *Tutors Guide: Basic Skills*. Darwin: Aboriginal Health Worker Training Programme.

————. 1995a. *The Aboriginal and Torres Strait Islander Guide to Healthy Eating: Educator's Resource*. Darwin: Northern Territory Government.

————. 1995b. *Food for Thought in Rural Aboriginal Communities: An Information Booklet for Remote Northern Territory Store Managers*. Darwin: Northern Territory Department of Health and Community Services.

————. 1996. *NT Aboriginal Health Policy 1996*. Darwin: Territory Health Services.

————. 1998a. *The Aboriginal and Torres Strait Islander Guide to Healthy Eating: Flyer and Poster*. Darwin: Northern Territory Government.

————. 1998b. *Annual Report*. Darwin: Territory Health Services.

————. 1998c. *National Aboriginal Health Performance Indicators, NT*. Darwin: Northern Territory Government.

————. 2002. *Keeping Fit, Keeping Healthy, Keeping Strong*. Darwin: Northern Territory Government.

————. 2004. *Annual Report 2003–2004*. Darwin: Northern Territory Government.

————. 2005. *Aboriginal Health and Families: A Five Year Framework for Action*. Darwin: Department of Health and Community Services.

————. 2007. *Annual Report 2006–2007*. Casuarina, NT: Department of Health and Community Services.

————. 2008a. *Annual Report 2007–2008*. Casuarina, N.T.: Department of Health and Community Services.

————. 2008b. *Northern Territory Market Basket Survey 2008*. Darwin: Department of Health and Families.

Northern Territory Government. 1997. *Northern Territory Government Submission to the House of Representatives Standing Committee on Family and Community Affairs Inquiry into Indigenous Health*. Darwin: Northern Territory Government.

————. 2007. *Closing the Gap of Indigenous Disadvantage: A Generational Plan of Action.*" Darwin: Northern Territory Government.

O'Brien, Patty. 1998. "The Gaze of the Ghosts: European Images of Aboriginal Women in New South Wales and Port Phillip 1800–1850." In *Maps, Dreams, History: Race and Representation in Australia*, edited by J. Kociumbas and R. Glover, 313–400. Sydney: University of Sydney Press.

O'Dea, Kerin. 1983. "Ten Diabetics Go Bush." *The Aboriginal Health Worker* 7 (4): 26–29.

————. 1985. "Relationship between Lifestyle-Changes and Health in Aborigines." In *Alcohol and Drug Use in a Changing Society: Proceedings of the 2nd National Drug Institute, Darwin, Northern Territory, Australia, 1985*, edited by K. Larkins, D. McDonald and C. Watson, 96–102. Canberra: National Drug Institute.

O'Mara, Peter. 2010. "Health Impacts of the Northern Territory Intervention." *Medical Journal of Australia* 192 (10): 546–8.

Opie, Tessa, Sue Lenthall, Maureen Dollard, John Wakerman, Martha MacLeod, Sabina Knight, Sandra Dunn, and Greg Rickard. 2010. "Trends in Workplace Violence in the Remote Area Nursing Workforce." *Australian Journal of Advanced Nursing* 27 (4): 18–23.

Oropeza, Laura. 2002. *Clinicians Guide: Working with Native Americans Living with HIV*. Oakland, CA: National Native American AIDS Prevention Center.

Paine, Robert. 1977. "The Path to Welfare Colonialism." In *The White Arctic: Anthropological Essays on Tutelage and Ethnicity*, edited by R. Paine, 3–28. St. John: Memorial University of Newfoundland.

Paradies, Yin. 2007. "Racism." In *Social Determinants of Indigenous Health*, edited by B. Carson, 65–79. Crows Nest, N.S.W.: Allen & Unwin.

Peile, Anthony Rex. 1997. *Body and Soul: An Aboriginal View*. Carlisle, W.A.: Hesperian Press.

Peterson, Nicolas. 1969. "Secular and Ritual Links: Two Basic Opposed Principles of Australian Social Organization as Illustrated by Walbiri Ethnography." *Mankind* 7:27–35.

————. 1991. "Cash, Commoditisation and Authenticity: When Do Aboriginal People Stop Being Hunter-Gatherers." In *Cash, Commoditisation and Changing Foragers*, edited by N. Peterson and T. Matsuyama, 67–90. Osaka: National Museum of Ethnology.

————. 1993. "Demand Sharing: Reciprocity and the Pressure for Generosity among Foragers." *American Anthropologist* 95 (4): 860–74.

————. 1998. "Welfare Colonialism and Citizenship: Politics, Economics and Agency." In *Citizenship and Indigenous Australians*, edited by N. Peterson and W. Sanders, 101–17. Cambridge: Cambridge University Press.

————. 1999. "Hunter-Gatherers in First World Nation States: Bringing Anthropology Home." *Bulletin of the National Museum of Ethnology* 23 (4): 847–61.

————. 2010. "Culture Crisis: Anthropology and Politics in Aboriginal Australia." In *Culture Crisis: Anthropology and Politics in Aboriginal Australia*, edited by J. Altman and M. Hinkson, 248–58. Sydney: University of New South Wales.

Peterson, Nicolas, Patrick McConvell, Steven Wild, and Rod Hagen. 1978. *A Claim to Areas of Traditional Land by the Warlpiri and Kartangarurru-Kurintji*. Alice Springs: Central Land Council.

Peterson, Nicolas, and John Taylor. 2003. "The Modernising of the Indigenous Domestic Moral Economy: Kinship, Accumulation and Household Composition." *The Asia Pacific Journal of Anthropology* 4 (1&2): 105–22.

Phillips, H. 1990. "The Origin of the Public Health Act of 1919." *South African Medical Journal* 77 (10): 531–2.

Pink, Brian, and Penny Allbon. 2008. *The Health and Welfare of Australia's Aboriginal and Torres Strait Islander Peoples 2008*. Canberra: Australian Bureau of Statistics.

Poirier, S. 2005. *A World of Relationships: Itineraries, Dreams, and Events in the Australian Western Desert*. Toronto: Toronto University Press.

Povenelli, Elizabeth A. 1993. *Labor's Lot: The Power, History, and Culture of Aboriginal Action*. Chicago: University of Chicago Press.

————. 2010. "Indigenous Politics in Late Liberalism." In *Culture Crisis: Anthropology and Politics in Aboriginal Australia*, edited by J. Altman and M. Hinkson, 17–31. Sydney: University of New South Wales Press.

Press, Irwin. 1980. "Problems in the Definition and Classification of Medical Systems." *Social Science and Medicine* 14B:45–57.

Public Accounts Committee. 1996. *Report on the Provision of Health Service to Aboriginal Communities in the Northern Territory*. Darwin: Northern Territory Government.

Radcliffe-Brown, A. R. 1926. "The Rainbow Serpent Myth of Australia." *The Journal of the Royal Anthropological Institute of Great Britain and Ireland* 56:19–25.

Reid, Janice, ed. 1982. *Body, Land, and Spirit: Health and Healing in Aboriginal Society*. St. Lucia: University of Queensland Press.

Reid, Janice. 1983. *Sorcerers and Healing Spirits: Continuity and Change in an Aboriginal Medical System*. Canberra: Australian National Press.

Reiser, S. J. 1985. "Responsibility for Personal Health: A Historical Perspective." *Journal of Medicine and Philosophy* 10 (1): 7–17.

Ring, Ian, and Ngaire Brown. 2002. "Indigenous Health: Chronically Inadequate Responses To Damning Statistics." *Medical Journal of Australia* 177 (11): 629–31.

Ritchie, Linda. 2001. "Empowerment and Australian Community Health Nurses' Work with Aboriginal Clients: The Sociopolitical Context." *Qualitative Health Research* 11 (2): 190–205.

Robins, Patricia. 1996. "Context of Silence: Violence and the Remote Area Nurse." In *Aboriginal Health: Social and Cultural Transitions*, edited by G. Robinson, 129–35. Darwin: Northern Territory University Press.

Roheim, Geza. 1974. *Children of the Desert*. New York: Basic Books.

Rose, Deborah Bird. 1991. *Hidden Histories: Black Stories from Victoria River Downs, Humbert River, and Wave Hill Stations*. Canberra: Aboriginal Studies Press.

———. 1992. *Dingo Makes Us Human: Life and Land in an Australian Aboriginal Culture*. Cambridge: Cambridge University Press.

Rouse, Carolyn. 2010. "Patient and Practitioner Noncompliance: Rationing, Therapeutic Uncertainty, and the Missing Conversation." *Anthropology & Medicine* 17 (2): 187–200.

Rowse, Tim. 1998. *White Flour, White Power: From Rations to Citizenship in Central Australia*. Cambridge: Cambridge University Press.

Rowse, Tim, David Scrimgeour, Sabrina Knight, and David Thomas. 1994. "Food-Purchasing Behaviour in an Aboriginal Community: 1: Results of a Survey." *Australian Journal of Public Health* 18 (1): 63–66.

Roy, Bernard. 2006. "Diabetes and Identity: Changes in the Food Habits of the Innu." In *Indigenous People and Diabetes: Community Empowerment and Wellness*, edited by M. L. Ferreira and G. C. Lang, 167–86. Durham, NC: Carolina Academic Press.

Russell, Beth J., Andrew V. White, Jonathan Newbury, Carmel Hattch, Jennie Thurley, and Anne B. Chang. 2004. "Evaluation of Hospitalisation for Indigenous children with Malnutrition Living in Central Australia." *Australian Journal of Rural Health* 12:187–91.

Saethre, Eirik. 2005. "Nutrition, Economics, and Food Distribution in an Australian Aboriginal Community." *Anthropological Forum* 15 (2): 151–69.

———. 2007a. "Close Encounters: UFO Beliefs in Remote Aboriginal Australia." *Journal of the Royal Anthropological Institute (N.S.)* 13 (4): 901–15.

————. 2007b. "Conflicting Traditions, Concurrent Treatment: Medical Pluralism in Remote Aboriginal Australia." *Oceania* 77:95–110.

————. 2007c. "UFOs, Otherness, and Belonging: Identity in Remote Aboriginal Australia." *Social Identities* 13 (2): 217–33.

Saethre, Eirik J., and Jonathan Stadler. 2009. "A Tale of Two 'Cultures': HIV/AIDS Risk Narratives in South Africa." *Medical Anthropology* 28 (3): 268–84.

Saggers, Sherry, and Dennis Gray. 1991. *Aboriginal Health and Society: The Traditional and Contemporary Aboriginal Struggle for Better Health*. Sydney: Allen and Unwin.

Sansom, Basil. 1980. *The Camp at Wallaby Cross: Aboriginal Fringe Dwellers in Darwin*. Canberra: Australian Institute of Aboriginal Studies.

Santiago-Irizarry, Vilma. 2001. *Medicalizing Ethnicity: The Construction of Latino Identity in a Psychiatric Setting*. Ithaca, NY: Cornell University Press.

Scheppers, Emmanuel, Els van Dongen, Jos Dekker, Jan Geertzen, and Joost Dekker. 2006. "Potential Barriers to the Use of Health Services among Ethnic Minorities: A Review." *Family Practice* 23 (3): 325–48.

Schwarz, Carolyn. 2010a. "Carrying the Cross, Caring for Kin: The Everyday Life of Charismatic Christianity in Remote Aboriginal Australia." *Oceania* 80:58–77.

————. 2010b. "Sick Again, Well Again: Sorcery, Christianity and Kinship in Northern Aboriginal Australia." *Anthropological Forum* 20 (1): 61–81.

Scrimgeour, D., T. Rowse, and A. Lucas. 1997. *Too Much Sweet: The Social Relations of Diabetes in Central Australia*. Alice Springs: Menzies School of Health Research.

Sevo, Goran. 2003. *Multidimensional Assessment of Health and Functional Status of Older Aboriginal Australians* from Katherine and Lajamanu N.T. PhD diss., Department of Archaeology and Anthropology, Australian National University, Canberra.

Sharp, Ian. 1966. "Report on the Present Wage Position of Aborigines in the Northern Territory." In *Aborigines in the Economy*, edited by I. Sharp and C. M. Tatz, 145–73. Brisbane: Jacaranda Press.

Shaw, Susan J., and Julie Armin. 2011. "The Ethical Self-Fashioning of Physicians and Health Care Systems in Culturally Appropriate Health Care." *Culture, Medicine and Psychiatry* 35:236–61.

Skov, Steven. 1994. "Traditional Concepts of Health among Aboriginal People." *Central Australian Rural Practitioners Newsletter* 19:15–21.

Soong, Foong San. 1981. *Developing the Role of Primary Health Workers (Aboriginal) in the Northern Territory*. Darwin: Northern Territory Department of Health.

Spencer, Baldwin, and Francis J. Gillen. 1904. *Northern Tribes of Central Australia*. London: Macmillan.

Stewart, Ian. 1997. *Research into the Cost, Availability and Preferences for Fresh Food Compared with Convenience Food.* Canberra: Roy Morgan Research Centre.

Stillwaggon, Eileen. 2003. "Racial Metaphors: Interpreting Sex and AIDS in Africa." *Development and Change* 34 (5): 809–32.

Stocking, G. W. 1982. *Race, Culture, and Evolution: Essays in the History of Anthropology.* Chicago: University of Chicago Press.

Sullivan, Patrick. 2005. "Searching for the Intercultural, Searching for the Culture." *Oceania* 75 (3): 183–94.

———. 2006. "Introduction: Culture without Cultures—the Culture Effect." *The Australian Journal of Anthropology* 17 (3): 253–64.

Sutton, Peter. 2005. "The Politicisation of Disease and the Disease of Politicisation: Causal Theories and the Indigenous Health Differential." Paper read at National Rural Health Conference, at Alice Springs, Northern Territory.

———. 2009. *The Politics of Suffering: Indigenous Australia and the End of the Liberal Consensus.* Melbourne: Melbourne University Press.

Tatz, Colin. 1972. "The Politics of Aboriginal Health." Paper read at National Seminar on Aboriginal Health Services, at Sydney.

Taylor, Janelle S. 2003. "Confronting 'Culture' in Medicine's 'Culture of No Culture.'" *Academic Medicine* 78 (6): 555–9.

Taylor, John. 1977. "Murri Doctor or Nursing Sister? Part I." *The Aboriginal Health Worker* 1 (4): 27–39.

———. 1978. "Murri Doctor or Nursing Sister? Part II: The Nurses' Point of View." *The Aboriginal Health Worker* 2 (1): 37–46.

Taylor, Julie J. 2007. "Assisting or Compromising Intervention? The Concept of 'Culture' in Biomedical and Social Research on HIV/AIDS." *Social Science and Medicine* 64:965–75.

Taylor, Kerry. 1997. *Aboriginal Health Workers at Alice Springs Hospital: A Pilot Project to Evaluate Alternative Models of Practice for Aboriginal Health Workers.* Alice Springs: Territory Health Services.

Thomas, David Piers. 2004. *Reading Doctor's Writing: Race, Politics, and Power in Indigenous Health Research 1870–1969.* Canberra: Aboriginal Studies Press.

Thomas, David P., John R. Condon, Ian P. Anderson, Shu Q. Li, Stephen Halpin, Joan Cunningham, and Steven L. Guthridge. 2006. "Long-Term Trends in Indigenous Deaths from Chronic Diseases in the Northern Territory: A Foot on the Brake, a Foot on the Accelerator." *Medical Journal of Australia* 185 (3): 145–9.

Thomson, Neil. 1984. "Aboriginal Health and Health-Care." *Social Science and Medicine* 18 (11): 939–48.

Thomson, Neil, and Bruce English. 1992. "Development of the National Aboriginal Health Strategy." *Aboriginal Health Information Bulletin* 17 (May): 22–30.

Tom-Orme, Lillian. 1993. "Traditional Beliefs and Attitudes about Diabetes among Navajos and Utes." In *Diabetes as a Disease of Civilization: The Impact of Culture Change on Indigenous Peoples*, edited by J. R. Joe and R. S. Young, 271–91. New York: Walter de Gruyter and Co.

Tonkinson, Myrna. 1982. "The Mabarn and the Hospital: The Selection of Treatment in a Remote Aboriginal Community." In *Body, Land and Spirit: Health and Healing in Aboriginal Society*, edited by J. Reid, 225–41. St. Lucia: University of Queensland Press.

Tonkinson, Robert. 1978. *The Mardudjara Aborigines: Living the Dream in Australia's Desert*. New York: Holt, Rinehart and Winston.

Torr, Sally. 1988. "Aboriginal Views of Aboriginal Health Workers." *The Aboriginal Health Worker* 12 (1): 26–36.

Tregenza, John, and Kathy Abbot. 1995. *Rhetoric and Reality: Perceptions of the Roles of Aboriginal Health Workers in Central Australia*. Alice Springs: Central Australian Aboriginal Congress.

Treichler, Paula. 1999. *How to Have Theory in an Epidemic*. Durham, NC: Duke University Press.

Trewin, Dennis. 2006. *National Aboriginal and Torres Strait Islander Survey, Australia 2004–05*. Canberra: Australian Bureau of Statistics.

Trigger, David. 1992. *Whitefella Comin': Aboriginal Responses to Colonialism in Northern Australia*. Cambridge: Cambridge University Press.

Tyler, William. 1992. "Crosslines: Aboriginality, Postmodernity and the Australian State." *Humanity and Society* 18 (1): 4–21.

———. 1993. "Postmodernity and the Aboriginal Condition: The Cultural Dilemmas of Contemporary Policy." *Australia and New Zealand Journal of Sociology* 29 (3): 322–42.

United Nations. 2007. *World Population Prospects: The 2006 Revision*. New York: United Nations Department of Economic and Social Affairs, Population Division.

Walker, David. 1997/98. "Climate, Civilization and Character in Australia, 1880–1940." *Australian Cultural History* 16:77–95.

Wayland, Coral. 2004. "The Failure of Pharmaceuticals and the Power of Plants: Medicinal Discourse as a Critique of Modernity in the Amazon." *Social Science and Medicine* 58:2409–19.

Welsch, Robert. 1991. "Traditional Medicine and Western Medical Options among the Nigerum of Papua New Guinea." In *The Anthropology of Medicine: From Culture to Method*, edited by L. Romanucci-Ross, D. Moerman and L. Tancredi, 32–55. New York: Bergin & Garvey.

Whitmarsh, Ian. 2008. *Biomedical Ambiguity: Race, Asthma, and the Contested Meaning of Genetic Research in the Caribbean*. Ithaca, NY: Cornell University Press.

Whyte, Susan Reynolds, Sjaak van der Geest, and Anita Hardon. 2002. *The Social Lives of Medicines*. Cambridge: Cambridge University Press.

Wikler, D. 1987. "Who Should Be Blamed for Being Sick?" *Health Education Quarterly* 14 (1): 11–25.

Wild, Stephen. 1975. *Walbiri Music and Dance in their Social and Cultural Nexus*. PhD diss., Indiana University.

Willis, Eileen. 1985. *Servant of Two Masters: A Study of an Aboriginal Health Worker Literacy Program in the Southern Region of the Northern Territory*. M.Ed. thesis, Department of Education, University of New England, Armidale, N.S.W.

Worboys, Michael. 1990. "Manson, Ross and Colonial Medical Policy: Tropical Medicine in London and Liverpool, 1899–1914." In *Disease, Medicine and Empire: Perspectives on Western Medicine and the Experience of European Expansion*, edited by R. Macleod and M. Lewis, 21–37. New York: Routledge.

World Health Organization. 1946. *Preamble to the Constitution of the World Health Organization as Adopted by the International Health Conference*, New York, 19–22 June, 1946. New York: World Health Organization.

———. 2004. *The World Medicines Situation*. Geneva: World Health Organization.

Wright, J. 1981. *The Cry for the Dead*. Oxford: Oxford University Press.

Yarwood, A. T. 1991. "Sir Raphael Cilento and the White Man in the Tropics." In *Health and Healing in Tropical Australia and Papua New Guinea*, edited by R. Macleod and D. Denoon, 47–63. Townsville, QLD: James Cook University Press.

Young, Elspeth. 1995. *Third World in the First: Development and Indigenous People*. London: Routledge.

Zhao, Yuejen, and Karen Dempsey. 2006. "Causes of Inequality in Life Expectancy between Indigenous and Non-Indigenous People in the Northern Territory, 1981–2000: A Decomposition Analysis." *Medical Journal of Australia* 184 (10): 490–4.

Zhao, Yuejen, Christine Connors, Jo Wright, Steve Guthridge, and Ross Bailie. 2008. "Estimating Chronic Disease Prevalence among the Remote Aboriginal Population of the Northern Territory using Multiple Data Sources." *Australian and New Zealand Journal of Public Health* 32 (4): 307–13.

Zhao, Yuejen, Steve Guthridge, Anne Mangus, and Theo Vos. 2004. "Burden of Disease and Injury in Aboriginal and Non-Aboriginal Populations of the Northern Territory." *Medical Journal of Australia* 180:498–502.

Index